FRIENDS
OF ACPL

D1558936

BOYS
into
MEN

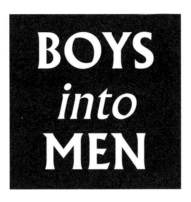

BOYS into MEN

Staying Healthy through the Teen Years

Mark A. Goldstein, M.D.
and Myrna Chandler Goldstein

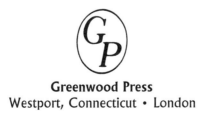

Greenwood Press
Westport, Connecticut • London

Library of Congress Cataloging-in-Publication Data

Goldstein, Mark A. (Mark Allan), 1947–
     Boys into men : staying healthy through the teen years / by Mark A. Goldstein
and Myrna Chandler Goldstein.
         p.   cm.
     Includes bibliographical references and index.
     ISBN 0–313–30966–3 (alk. paper)
     1. Adolescent boys—Health and hygiene.   2. Adolescent boys—Psychology.
     3. Teenage boys—Health and hygiene.   I. Goldstein, Myrna Chandler, 1948–
     II. Title.
     RA777.2.G65   2000
     613'.04233—dc21   00–021045

British Library Cataloguing in Publication Data is available.

Library of Congress Catalog Card Number: 00–021045
ISBN: 0–313–30966–3

First published in 2000

Greenwood Press, 88 Post Road West, Westport, CT 06881
An imprint of Greenwood Publishing Group, Inc.
www.greenwood.com

Printed in the United States of America

The paper used in this book complies with the
Permanent Paper Standard issued by the National
Information Standards Organization (Z39.48–1984).

10 9 8 7 6 5 4 3 2 1

The information in this book should not be used as a substitute for medical care and the
advice of a physician. Any application of the treatments set forth in this book is at the
reader's sole discretion and neither the author nor the publisher assumes any responsibility
or liability therefor.

Copyright Acknowledgments

Illustrations courtesy of Matthew Roth.

Material quoted from Richard M. Schwartzstein, M.D., "The Wellesley Townsman," October 23, 1997 used by permission.

To all the boys who have entrusted their care to me,
shared their most intimate concerns,
and inspired me to write this book

About the Illustrator: Matthew Roth has been a quadriplegic since an accident during his own adolescence. He drew all the illustrations for this volume using his mouth and lips.

Contents

Acknowledgments   ix

Introduction   xi

1   Healthcare Issues   1

2   Epidemiology and Statistics   7

3   Physical and Emotional Growth and Development   15

4   General Nutrition and Sports Nutrition   25

5   Sexuality   45

6   Alcohol, Tobacco, and Drugs   61

7   Sports Injuries and Sports Medicine   75

8   Adolescent Medical Concerns and Practices   95

9   Outdoor and Wilderness Health   115

10 Life Issues   133

11 Behavior, Mental and Emotional Health Issues   151

12 Cross-Cultural Issues and Your Health   169

13 Issues for Gay Adolescents   173

14 Chronic Conditions   181

Index   189

Acknowledgments

When you teach your son, you teach your son's son.
Talmud, Kiddushin

I wish to thank my spouse and coauthor, Myrna Chandler Goldstein, for all of her assistance in reviewing and rewriting the manuscript. She has the talent to create readable material from my rambling and often incomprehensible writings. Without her enormous efforts, this book would not exist.

Emily Birch, our editor at the Greenwood Publishing Group, has been of immense help in reviewing the manuscript. Her objective review of the chapters and constructive comments have been invaluable.

Robert Masland, M.D., chief emeritus of the Adolescent Unit at the Children's Hospital in Boston, has been my mentor for many years. His understanding of the medical and psychological needs of adolescents has profoundly influenced my career. It is in large part because of Dr. Masland that I chose to specialize in adolescent medicine. He will always be my most cherished teacher and friend.

During the year in which I taught adolescent medicine to Justine Julia Larson and Laura Michelle Gottlieb, two Harvard Medical School students, they reviewed portions of the manuscript. I very much appreciate Justine's sensitivity to the psychosocial issues of boys, and Laura's constructive comments on risky behaviors in teens. From their sincere interest in the issues of teens, it is quite evident that they will soon become outstanding, caring, and sensitive physicians.

I thank psychiatrist Gregory Gale, M.D., for his critical reading of sections of the manuscript. His comments presented important insights and caused me to rethink several issues.

You may have already noted the many illustrations that fill this book. They are the work of Matthew Roth, who has been a quadriplegic since a tragic accident in his mid-adolescence. A few years ago, Myrna interviewed Matthew for a newspaper article. Later, she wrote a magazine piece on him. Shortly after we signed our contract with Greenwood, we asked Emily if Matthew could be our illustrator. She heartedly agreed. Using a pencil and the movement of his lips, Matthew has produced thoughtful, artistic, and sensitive drawings.

And, finally, I wish to thank the thousands of boys who have entrusted their medical care to me. Your stories inspired me to write this book. What I have learned from you has made me a better physician, and I have been able to pass that knowledge along to my students. I am forever grateful.

Introduction

The question was not uncommon. I had heard it many times. Just as I was about to complete the physical exam of an 18-year-old male patient, the patient turned to me and said, "By the way, I'm leaving for college next week. How can I protect myself from getting a sexually transmitted disease?" He had a specific question, and, as his physician, I should be there to provide the appropriate answers. So, we talked about the methods males may use to avoid contracting these diseases, including knowing your partner, being monogamous, using condoms, and practicing abstinence.

I had cared for this patient since his birth and had helped him acquire the skills to take control of his medical care. During his adolescent years, without the presence of his parents in the room, we had discussed a multitude of issues important to him and other males. He had asked me about his developing body, how tall he would be, how to become more muscular, and why he seemed to have a slight breast development. We had talked about his potential exposure to alcohol and marijuana and how to react when his friends asked him to join in risky behaviors. He also expressed concern about dealing with his parents—especially how he could grow increasingly independent while retaining strong relationships with his family members. The last year of high school, we dealt with the added stress of applying to college. I valued the strength of our doctor/patient relationship, and I looked forward to his continued visits during his college years and for a few years thereafter.

That is the role of a physician who specializes in adolescent medicine. We help adolescents monitor their physical, psychological, and social well-being as they make the transition into healthy, self-sufficient young adults.

Adolescence is generally defined as the period between ages 12 and 21. It is a time when the body and mind undergo tremendous changes— from that of a concrete-thinking child to that of an independent and mature adult. I generally divide adolescence into three time frames— early, ages 12 to 14, which correlates with middle school; mid-adolescence, ages 15 to 18, corresponding to the high school years; and late adolescence, ages 19 to 21, when young adults are completing higher education, military service, and/or working. In my training and practice, I see adolescents through young adulthood, which is defined as up to age 25. Each of these time frames involves substantial physical, psycho-logical, and social issues that male adolescents need to address. Many of these issues could present serious obstacles to the successful completion of adolescence.

Fortunately, many physicians and other healthcare providers have dis-cussed the healthcare issues of female adolescents. There is a plethora of books available on the topic. Moreover, teenage girls seek the advice of their peers and their healthcare professionals more often than boys. In many instances, they talk to their parents more readily than boys do.

While boys are intensely interested in their bodies, they do not talk about this concern with their parents or peers. They worry about aches, pains, and acne, but will not broach the subject with others, unless placed in the proper environment. As a physician who has specialized in the care of adolescents for 23 years, I try to create an atmosphere that en-courages and welcomes questions.

In my practice of adolescent medicine, I try to teach teens to assume responsibility for their medical care. My goal is for each high school–graduating senior to be comfortable with recognizing illness, telephoning a physician, and continuing a responsible doctor/patient relationship. With my patients, I discuss confidentiality, routine medical care, signifi-cant symptoms, and checking one's body for signs of illness. By the time he leaves home, every teenage male should be responsible for his medi-cal care.

Given the correct factual medical information, adolescent boys will be able to make informed and, hopefully, safe decisions as they grow into young adults. But they must have clear answers to their questions, even those they are afraid to ask. On countless occasions, I have seen boys between the ages of 12 and 14 who had small breast development. I always point this out as a stage of normal male development. Invariably, I observe a sense of great relief. At that state of adolescence, the boys feel that there is something terribly wrong. Perhaps it is a indicator of incipient feminine traits or serious illness, such as a malignant breast tumor. While information offered during the physical exam is useful, a written resource would also be valuable.

Recently, I saw a male adolescent patient who just completed his freshman year at a highly competitive university. At one point, he mentioned that, during a particularly stressful time, he binged on alcohol. He blacked out and was rushed by ambulance to the hospital. We used that experience to discuss the appropriate consumption of alcohol for an 18-year-old who is legally under age, including the possible deadly consequences of dangerous drinking. The brightest boys may succumb to risky behavior. All adolescent males need more information on risky behaviors, such as substance abuse, sexuality, and violence.

Adolescence is filled with emotional upheavals. Aside from the physical, emotional and social changes that occur, you may face other stresses. Marriages fall apart, and parents divorce. Social relations break down, and you have to endure failures in school and sports. Some teens develop chronic illnesses. A number of my patients have become depressed or anxious; some have developed antisocial or violent behaviors. A few have been diagnosed with Attention Deficit Disorder, a disorder characterized by a lessened ability to focus on certain activities and treatable with medication. Teens need to know about these potential problems.

This volume is meant to provide information for male teens who do not feel comfortable talking with others about their health concerns. Arranged topically, each of the chapters covers a different aspect of both mind and body concerns from sports injuries, to sexuality, to substance use and abuse. In this book male teens can get straight answers to their questions about their growing minds and bodies. From there, they can consult with their own physicians if they have further questions or concerns.

I have found nothing more gratifying than helping adolescent males through these difficult years. I have seen thousands of male patients successfully weather adolescence, graduate from college, and begin to build their careers. It has been said—and I do believe—that a doctor's best teachers are his patients. In this book I will share many of the experiences of my male patients and how we worked together to solve their problems. Let us hope that we all learn from this process.

1

Healthcare Issues

The field of adolescent medicine was born in the early 1950s at the Boston Children's Hospital. Prior to that, children up to the age of 12 were cared for by pediatricians; after 12, they were seen by general practitioners or internists. Fortunately, physicians at the Children's Hospital realized that adolescents face unique physical, emotional, social, and mental health issues. There is now a board-certifiable medical specialty devoted to adolescence.

Many insurance plans require you to have a primary care physician. If you're an adolescent, this physician should be sensitive to your particular needs. If you have a medical school nearby, you could contact its division of adolescent medicine for names of physicians who offer adolescent medical care. Well-trained specialists in adolescent medicine may address a range of concerns, including sports problems, skin problems, sexually transmitted diseases, and birth control. When necessary, they can refer you to specialists.

Naturally, you would be seeking medical care from a practitioner who is qualified, concerned, and empathetic. Good care may be obtained from a variety of practitioners who may or may not be adolescent medicine specialists or who may not even have a medical degree. You need a comfortable working relationship with a practitioner. You must be able to communicate with your provider, and the provider must be able to communicate with you.

Communication means being able to share your concerns with your provider. Some things, such as a pimple, may seem trivial to others. But they are not trivial to you, and your provider should take them seriously. A sensitive provider will understand this. And you should also be able to discuss with your provider more personal issues as well, such as problems with your parents and friends or the possibility that you may have contracted a sexually transmitted disease. Studies have shown that most adolescent males would like to discuss exercise, growth, sexually transmitted diseases, substance abuse, contraception, school issues, and acne with their healthcare providers.

Recently, I saw a 17-year-old male who was very concerned about the possibility that he had acquired HIV from a single sexual experience in which he had not used a condom. After talking about the risks and benefits of the HIV test, we arranged for him to be tested. We repeated it three months later. Both tests were negative. He felt comfortable discussing the issue with me because he knew that any test results would not be shared with his parents, unless he signed a special release form.

While you need a provider who listens to you, you should also listen to the provider. Establish a communication link—whether by telephone, letter, or e-mail. Increasingly, e-mail is becoming an efficient way to get quick answers to your questions.

Adolescent healthcare is available in many settings, some of which will depend on your health insurance. The traditional private office setting is common. However, there are very few physicians who practice nothing but adolescent medicine in a private office. You may find a responsive doctor in neighborhood health clinics, hospital-based adolescent units, free clinics, school-based clinics, and HMOs. There are even job-based clinics, such as Job Corps.

To some degree, the setting will dictate the type of providers you will see. Private offices are generally staffed by physicians. Clinics offer both physicians and nonphysician providers. Hospital-based adolescent units have trainees, such as medical students, residents, and fellows as well as staff physicians. Physicians and nonphysicians work for HMOs. The setting itself does not determine the appropriateness of the care. The provider-patient relationship is the key determinant.

In selecting a practitioner for your care, consider the following:

- Is the provider competent, caring, communicative, and understanding of male adolescent problems?
- Is the provider and his or her staff interested and committed to adolescents?
- Is the provider nonjudgmental and flexible?
- Are the hours convenient for you? The best hours for adolescents are usually late afternoon into the evening.
- Is the setting accessible?
- Will you have time alone with your provider to talk?

You should know how your provider feels about confidentiality. Confidentiality means that he or she will not reveal information to another

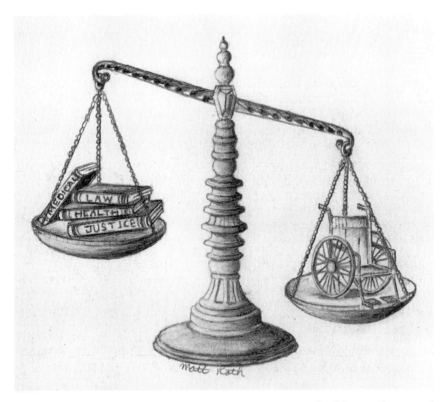

The law comes into play when it comes to minors getting healthcare. Courts and state laws have defined categories of adolescents who may give their own permission for their medical care.

party that you have shared privately. Most parents accept the fact that their sons will have a confidential relationship with their medical providers, especially if their sons are 14 years old or older. But there are a few exceptions to the confidentiality rule. In case of a serious risk to your life, your medical provider can share your personal information with your parents. And many sexually transmitted diseases must be reported to a state agency (but not to your parents). You should know that it is necessary for you or your parents to give consent for your medical care and procedures. With many aspects of your healthcare, you probably feel comfortable having your parents give permission. But sometimes you may not want them to be aware of a medical issue. Still, approval must be obtained. Every state now allows minors to consent for treatment of sexually transmitted diseases, emergencies, drug abuse, and contraception.

Additionally, courts and state laws have defined categories of adolescents who may give permission for their own medical care. Each state has its own provisions, but the following are common categories of minors who may consent to their own medical care:

- **Emancipated minors**: Adolescents under the age of 18 who are married or a parent or who are serving in the armed services or live separate from their parents and manage their own financial affairs.
- **Mature minors**: Adolescents, generally between the ages of 14 and 18, who, in the judgment of the physician can understand the risks and benefits of medical treatments.

While these categories of adolescents may consent to medical care, most states will also require a parent to sign an informed consent form for surgery involving adolescents under the age of 18.

TAKING CHARGE OF YOUR HEALTH

Your first visit to an adolescent medicine healthcare provider usually includes an oral and/or written history. Occasionally, a parent may contribute to this background review. You will be asked if you have any medical concerns. Many male teens are reluctant to acknowledge these kinds of concerns. An experienced provider should find ways to make you comfortable.

The provider will probably question you about more sensitive issues, including sexuality, drug and tobacco use, alcohol, violence, stress, as well as family, school, and peer relationships. This is an opportunity to share your problems, in confidence, with the provider.

During the physical examination, your provider will look for medical conditions frequently seen in adolescents. A complete exam usually includes a check for sexually transmitted diseases, testicular problems, hernias, and pubertal development. While you will probably feel embarrassed, all teen males and adult males undergo similar examinations. If you feel uncomfortable, tell your provider.

After the exam, your provider will discuss the results and make recommendations. Depending on your age, your parent might be asked to listen. Most of my patients between the ages of 14 and 18 prefer to speak with me alone. Afterwards, with the patient present, I might speak briefly to the parent. Many of my teen patients come to their appointments without either parent. I particularly remember a patient I have known now for 20 years. I saw him in the hospital as a newborn. Around puberty, he decided that his mother should not come into the examining room. About two years later, he began coming alone. By the age of 16, he was conducting all of his medical care alone.

Although you may be able to manage your medical care without the

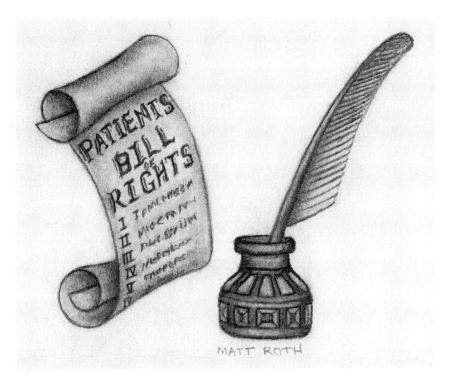

Teens are covered by the Patient's Bill of Rights.

assistance of your parents, if you do develop a serious problem, you should tell them about it. If you feel that you can't discuss your problem with a parent, ask your provider for guidance.

In order to monitor the growth, development, psychosocial health, and risky behaviors of their adolescent patients, most providers like to see them annually. This also allows for immunizations to be updated, especially those for hepatitis B, varicella, tetanus, and diphtheria. Unless you have a clinical problem, laboratory tests are generally not required each year. If you participate in sports, you are usually required to have an annual exam. Having a baseline check is good for you and your provider. If you become ill, your provider will already know your history. That may help him or her better manage your medical problems.

As you mature and take over more of your medical care, your provider will want you to become a responsible partner in your care. Compliance in adolescent medical care means that you follow instructions, such as obtaining tests, taking prescribed or recommended medication, and/or changing risky lifestyles. To encourage compliance, your provider may give you verbal and written instructions. He or she may also telephone or e-mail you and suggest that you return so that a condition may be monitored. When I first prescribe acne medications, I ask teens to return for monthly follow-ups. Within the bounds of confidentiality, the physician may request that others who are important to you, such as your parents and siblings, help you follow through on your healthcare.

As in other areas of life, when establishing a relationship with an adolescent medicine provider, cross-cultural and cross-gender issues must be considered. Some males prefer to see male providers; others do not care or would rather see a female provider. Some males prefer older providers; others want providers closer to their own age. Your provider may be of a different racial group or hold different ethical values. Clinical competency is not defined by age, gender, or ethnic or racial group. Your provider must be able to acknowledge and respect your background and values. If you feel that this is not the case, you should consider seeing another provider.

REFERENCE

Braverman, Paula K., and Victor C. Strasburger, editors. *Office-Based Adolescent Health Care, Adolescent Medicine: State of the Art Reviews*. Philadelphia: Henley & Belfus, February 1997.

2

Epidemiology and Statistics

To help you understand how to stay well, we need to review epidemiology and some statistics. Epidemiology is a field of science that deals with the relationships of factors that determine how often a disease, injury, or other process occurs in a human population.

Several years ago, one of my patients, who was only 14, was hit by a car while riding his bike. Unfortunately, he was not wearing a helmet. Thrown several feet, he hit his head, lost consciousness, and developed bleeding in his brain. Although he recovered, he suffered short-term memory loss, which persisted for some time and had a negative impact on his academic work. His neurologist believed that if he had been wearing a helmet, his injury could have been avoided.

The following data show percentages of teenage males who rarely or never wear a bicycle helmet while biking:

Grade 9	87.3%
Grade 10	86.2%
Grade 11	90.4%
Grade 12	89.8%
College	86.9%

Source: Centers for Disease Control 1998.

Thus, nine out of every 10 males rarely wear a bicycle helmet when biking, even though helmets have been shown to be effective in preventing head injury during an accident.

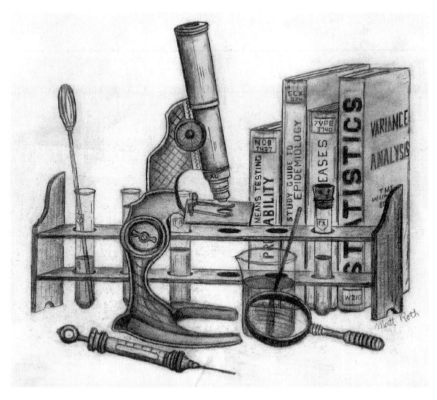

Scientists and doctors use many different methods to study the behavior of adolescents.

Many male teens behave in certain ways because they believe that their peers are acting in similar ways. Teens think that if they do not conform to the behavior of their peers, they are not cool. But you should know that what you think others are doing is not, necessarily, what's really going on.

Another type of potentially dangerous behavior is riding in a car with a driver who has been drinking alcohol. Every month of the year, but especially around prom time in June, you hear of teens killed in cars where the person behind the wheel had been drinking. Look at the statistics on males who ride with a driver who has been drinking:

Grade 9	31.8%
Grade 10	35.6%
Grade 11	42.9%
Grade 12	41.7%
College	39.7%

Source: Centers for Disease Control 1998.

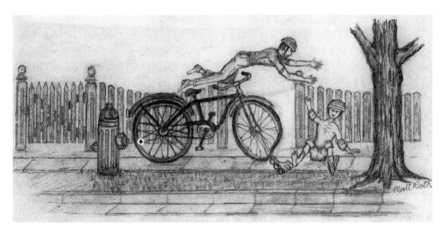

Even though helmets have been shown to be effective in preventing head injury during an accident, many teenagers don't wear them while biking and roller blading.

Never be a passenger in a car with a driver who has been drinking. It is important to select a designated driver in advance, and that person should refrain from drinking any alcoholic beverages.

Some teens behave in ways that bring about intentional injuries. For example, there has been much news coverage recently about teens who carry weapons to school. The Centers for Disease Control (CDC) publishes statistics on the percentages of male teens who carry a weapon (gun, club, or knife) to school:

Grade 9	33.2%
Grade 10	26.6%
Grade 11	28.8%
Grade 12	23.3%
College	7.5%

Source: Centers for Disease Control 1998.

These data show that at any time one-fourth to one-third of high school males have a weapon at school. One can only wonder why more high schools don't have stricter gun control measures, such as metal detectors and body searches.

About 4.5 percent of males attempt suicide in high school, and 1.7 percent try to kill themselves in college. Usually, a suicide victim has a major mental illness. Be sensitive to your own symptoms, or symptoms you see in your friends, that may be indicators of suicidal intentions. Seek help immediately. I know of teens who were able to intervene and prevent a peer from killing himself. Regrettably, I also know teens who were not sufficiently attuned to their friends' silent cries for help. When those friends later killed themselves, these students suffered enormous guilt.

You may think that most of your male friends in high school are sexually active. But you are wrong! The majority of boys in grades 9, 10, and 11 have never had sexual intercourse, and, of those who have had sexual intercourse at some point in their lifetime, up to 38 percent are not currently sexually active. The good news, to some extent, is that around 65 percent of males in high school who are sexually active used a condom during their last intercourse. The bad news is that 35 percent did not. When you do not use a condom, you place your partner at risk for pregnancy and/or sexually transmitted disease (STD), and you place yourself at risk of contracting a STD. The bottom line is that you should always use a condom.

It is wrong, immoral, and illegal to force someone to have sex against his or her will. According to the CDC, about 20 percent of college females have been forced to have sexual intercourse at least once. Invariably, males are forcing females to have sex. You almost never hear of females who force males to have sex.

The CDC contends that about 30 percent of high school males used drugs or alcohol before their last act of sexual intercourse. The dangers of combining drugs and/or alcohol with sex are obvious. You may force your partner to have sex against her or his will or you may forget to use a condom. By the way, under the influence of drugs and/or alcohol, sexual stimulation may be diminished.

I am sure that you agree that vigorous physical activity is good for your body and mind. The following are statistics from the CDC regarding the percentage of males who participate in vigorous physical activity, defined as activity that causes sweating and hard breathing, for at least 20 minutes three days a week:

Grade 9	78.7%
Grade 10	74.3%
Grade 11	68.9%
Grade 12	68.4%
College	45.0%

Source: Centers for Disease Control 1998.

To continue vigorous activity through adolescence and into adulthood, you need to find an activity you enjoy. Vigorous activity increases your endorphins, tones your muscles, relieves stresses, and can improve your self-image and outlook on life.

Let's look at some statistics regarding deaths from injuries for adolescents 15–19 years old in 1992:

Cause of Death	Death Rate Per 100,000 Population
Motor Vehicle Injury	28.2
Firearm Injury	26.2
Homicide	19.3
Suicide	10.8
Drowning	2.3

Source: National Center for Health Statistics.

Motor vehicle–related accidents are the most common cause of death from injuries for adolescents. And the most common type of fatal injury from a motor vehicle accident is a head injury. Head injury causes death in adolescents in about 60 percent of motor vehicle–occupant fatalities, 75 percent of pedestrian fatalities, and more than 60 percent of bicyclist fatalities. As you recall, about 90 percent of male teens do not wear bicycle helmets. Wouldn't that be an easy thing to do? Look at professional cyclists: They always wear helmets. And, obviously, wearing a seatbelt all the time would protect your head and other body injuries in a car crash.

When I was a volunteer ambulance attendant in medical school, my very first patient was a teen who drowned in a bathtub during a seizure. In about 50 percent of the cases of death from drowning, teens have been drinking alcohol. About 48 percent of the victims could not swim. Only a small percentage drown because of a seizure disorder.

From the data presented in this chapter, you should be able to see that you should not combine alcohol intake with swimming, driving, or sex. And never be a passenger in a car in which the driver has been drinking.

Looking at the causes of death in teens, you see that the number of deaths from violence is quite significant for males. Consider the following:

• Through mass media, teens are exposed to an incredible amount of violence.

• Viewers of violence in the mass media more readily accept aggressive attitudes and have increased aggressive behaviors.

• Viewers of violence become desensitized to violence and are more willing to accept violence directed at other individuals.

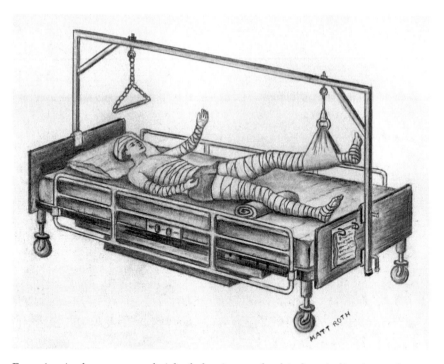

Engaging in dangerous and risky behavior can lead to hospitalization and even death.

- Films that depict women being raped can increase a male's belief that women desire rape and deserve sexual abuse.
- Explicit scenes of sexual violence against women in films appear to affect the attitudes of teens about rape and violence toward females.

Violence in the mass media is a major societal problem. But as a maturing adolescent male, you need to be able to control your thinking and emotions. Despite our violent environment, most of us pass through adolescence safely. During adolescence, one of your tasks is to learn how to view mass media violence with a critical eye. You need to recognize that violence may be portrayed in a totally unrealistic manner in the movies and on TV, and think of alternatives to a violent response to situations. You need to separate reality from fantasy.

REFERENCES

Centers for Disease Control and Prevention. "Youth Risk Behavior Surveillance National College Health Risk Behavior Survey—United States, 1995" November 14, 1997.

Centers for Disease Control and Prevention. "Youth Risk Behavior Surveillance—United States, 1997." August 14, 1998.

Christoffel, Katherine K, and Carol W Runyan, editors. *Adolescent Injuries: Epidemiology and Prevention, Adolescent Medicine: State of the Arts Reviews*. Philadelphia: Henley & Belfus, June 1995.

3

Physical and Emotional Growth and Development

During my fellowship training in adolescent medicine, one of my first patients was a 15-year-old male who had not started to develop. Because he would not undress in front of the other boys, he refused to participate in sports. Fortunately, he responded well to hormone treatment. And within a relatively brief period of time, his pubertal development began.

From the moment of conception until the end of life, your body and mind are in a constant state of change. Puberty is the four-year period when your body transitions from that of a child to that of an adult. Your mind also begins a process of change. During that time, which typically begins between the ages of 10 and 14, you experience major changes in appearance and your thinking process. In addition, you achieve the ability to reproduce and begin to develop adult emotions.

Complex hormonal relationships determine when the body begins puberty. Researchers have noted that boys at the beginning of the 21st century are entering puberty earlier than boys did 100 years ago. This is probably related to better nutrition and overall health.

Many of the events of puberty are triggered by the hypothalamus, an area in the brain that releases hormones. The hypothalamus is fairly quiet until you reach around age nine, when it starts to release pulsations of stimulating hormones. When these reach a certain level, they trigger an increased production of the sex hormones—follicle stimulating hormone (FSH) and luteinizing hormone (LH)—in the pituitary gland, which is also located in the brain. LH stimulates cells in your testicles to produce another hormone called testosterone. Testosterone production leads to many of the changes seen in male puberty, including the growth of genitals, development of hair in the armpits and pubic region, and the onset

Table 3.1
Sequence of Physical Changes during Puberty

	Average Male	Time After Puberty Begins
Enlargement of testicles starts	11–12 years	0
Early growth of pubic hair	12 years	.5 years
Enlargement of penis begins	13 years	1.5 years
Temporary breast development	13 years	1.5 years
Voice cracking begins	13 years	1.5 years
Growth spurt	13–14 years	2–2.5 years
Hair in the armpits appears	14 years	2.5 years
Ejaculation, wet dreams	14 years	2–2.5 years
Adult voice attained	15 years	3.5 years
Moustache begins to appear	15 years	3.5–4 years
Whiskers appear on cheeks	16 years	4–5 years

of a beard. In addition, it accelerates the growth of bones, increases the size of muscles, and enlarges the larynx. As the larynx enlarges, the voice begins to lower. Testosterone also causes sebaceous glands in the skin to secrete extra oil, which may lead to acne. And it initiates the sex drive.

Some males begin the process of puberty at age 10. Others do not begin until 14. Most begin between the ages of 10 and 14. Whenever it begins, puberty will cause significant changes in weight, height, and emotions. Table 3.1 outlines some of the changes that occur during puberty. The table is based on a male who begins puberty between the ages of 11 and 12.

Before puberty, the average boy grows about two inches a year. But about 2.5 years into puberty, there is a growth spurt in which the average boy grows about four inches in one year.

Figure 3.1 is a male growth chart published by the Centers for Disease Control. It represents data collected in the United States from a cross section of males who come from a variety of ethnic backgrounds and regions. There is a section for stature and another section for weight. On the X axis you will note age in years, and on the Y axis you will see inches or centimeters for the height chart and pounds or kilograms on the weight chart. There are seven curved lines beginning at age two and ending at age 18. These lines represent percentiles.

Let's look at the chart for boys age 14. If you take 100 boys who are age 14, the boy who is 70 inches in height is at the 95th percentile for height. This means he is taller than 94 percent of the boys his age, and shorter than 4 percent. The same system may be used for weight.

To find your place on the chart, plot your height in inches (for your age) on the X axis on the upper section of the chart. You can do the same for your weight in the lower section. Thus, if you are exactly 15

Figure 3.1
Boys: 2 to 18 Years (Stature for Age and Weight for Age)

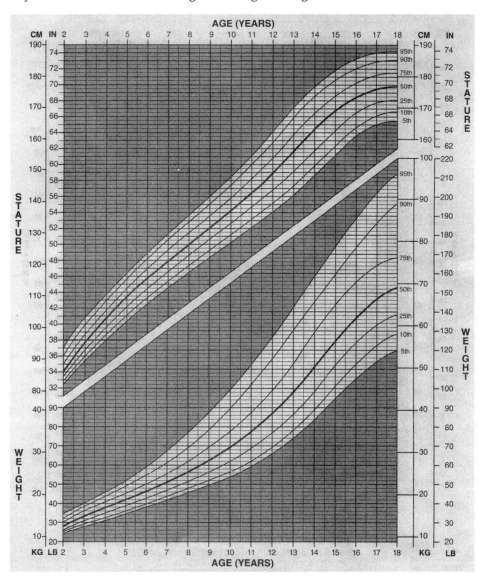

Source: Centers for Disease Control.

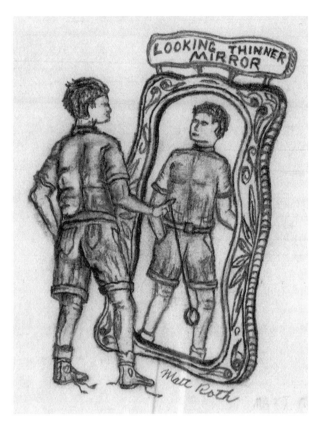

Most people do not have matching percentiles for their height and weight on the growth chart. More often, they fall somewhere in the range of 20% higher or lower than what the chart predicted.

years old, your current height is 67 inches, and you weigh 125 pounds, you are at the 50th percentile for height and weight. If you follow the 50th percentile dark line for height until age 18, you will see an ultimate height of 69.5 inches. This is an approximate prediction of your adult height. Although you will grow rapidly during your growth spurt, in the waning years of puberty, between 15 and 18 for most males, your height may only increase by about 2.5 inches.

From the growth chart you can approximate what your weight should be. Let's say you are 16.5 years old and are 71 inches tall. Your height is in the 75th percentile. Now look at the weight chart at age 16.5 and the 75th percentile. The weight corresponding to your height percentile is approximately 160 pounds. Most people do not have matching percentiles for their height and weight. More often, they fall somewhere in the range of 20 percent higher or lower than what the chart predicted. In this example, 20 percent of 160 pounds is 32 pounds. So, your weight could range from 128 pounds (160 minus 32) to 192 pounds (160 plus 32). At the lower end, you would be underweight for your height, and, at the upper end, you would probably be overweight for your height, unless you had a great deal of muscle mass.

Aside from your growth in height, your physical appearance during puberty is markedly affected by muscle mass. The increase in muscle mass caused by testosterone will occur in mid-puberty or about two years after the onset of puberty. It is then that the testosterone produced by your testicles increases. Your muscles actually increase in strength about a year after they increase in size. Weight training prior to puberty will have limited results. Until then, you do not have the circulating testosterone level to enlarge your muscles. Males continue to gain in muscle strength until the age of 25.

Your weight changes dramatically during puberty. Typically, when you are growing most rapidly in height and muscle mass, you will also be gaining the most weight. During the later part of puberty, the growth and muscle spurt, the average male gains 20 pounds a year. Of course, this rapid weight gain occurs for only a year or two.

Hormones cause about 70 percent of boys to experience some pubertal breast development. This usually recedes in a year or two, and there is no treatment for it since it is normal. If you are concerned about this, speak to your medical provider.

According to the Centers for Disease Control growth chart, the average (50th percentile) height for an 18-year-old-male is 69.5 inches. Those males above the 95th percentile for height at age 18 are 74 inches or taller. And those below the 5th percentile at age 18 are under 65 inches in height. Generally, very tall males do not suffer the psychological consequences of very short males. Shorter males sometimes feel self-conscious about their height, and their height may have a detrimental impact on their participation in sports and social life. On the other hand, shorter males have an advantage in certain sports such as gymnastics, soccer, tennis, and golf. But very tall males may also be disturbed about their height.

In the vast majority of cases, your adult height is a direct result of genetic makeup, which is inherited from your mother and father. However, I do recall one young teen who had a deficiency of growth hormone, which is very important for proper skeletal growth. Frequent injections of growth hormone, enabled him to gain extra height. But this therapy is used only when shortness is a result of hormonal problems. It is not prescribed when shortness is only a function of genes.

By the age of 14, the vast majority of boys have begun puberty. But about 3 percent have not. If you are in that group, your medical provider

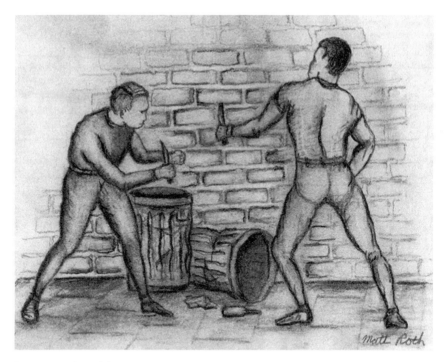

Society tends to blame aggressive male behaviors on "raging hormones." While it is true males are more likely to be physically aggressive than females, these tendencies actually stem from the male's upbringing, his peers, his place in society, and his values.

may want to do an evaluation. Most often, this is not the result of disease. Instead, it is caused by a "constitutional delay of puberty" or a delay in the mobilization of the hypothalamic-pituitary-testicle hormonal sequence described in the beginning of this chapter. Often, a biologically related relative has experienced a similar delay. Some boys may not begin to develop until they are 18. Nevertheless, once their development begins, it should proceed quite normally. During a medical evaluation, your provider will be able to rule out hormonal problems, nutritional issues, and systemic illnesses, and possibly prescribe treatment.

HORMONES AND BEHAVIOR

Society tends to blame aggressive adolescent male behaviors on "raging hormones." Is there any truth to that belief? It is true that males are more likely to be physically aggressive than females. They tend to play more combative sports or take more risks than females. But these activities begin at an early age, long before testosterone levels begin to rise.

Table 3.2
Sexuality Development

Early (12–14 years)
- begins to masturbate (experimenting with body)
- interested in privacy
- group activities and same sex friends

Middle (15–18 years)
- feelings of passion and tenderness in relationships
- movement toward heterosexuality or homosexuality
- frequent relationships

Late (19–21 years)
- sexual identity, whether heterosexual or homosexual, in place
- serious relationships may be forged
- ability to have tender and serious love

At least one study has shown a relationship between testosterone levels and aggressive activity in boys between the age of 15 and 17. However, aggressive behavior in male teens has not been shown in most studies to correlate with the teen's testosterone level. Aggressive behavior in a male teen is more likely due to his upbringing, his exposure to violence, and the type of society in which he lives. Young boys are simply more aggressive than young girls. Teenage boys with high testosterone levels are not necessarily aggressive; they may channel their energy into studies, music, or hobbies. What really underlies these aggressive tendencies are the male's upbringing, his peers, his place in society, and his values.

EMOTIONAL GROWTH AND DEVELOPMENT

Emotional growth and development may be divided into three categories: early (12–14 years, corresponding with middle school), middle (15–18 years, corresponding with high school), and late (19–21, corresponding with college). Tables 3.2, 3.3, and 3.4 examine three areas of emotional development and track them through early, middle, and late adolescence.

Emotional growth and development do not, necessarily, take place at the same time or pace as physical growth. You may be far advanced in goal-oriented behavior and, yet, still be at the beginning of physical development. Some boys have a physically normal development but are emotionally less mature. These boys may require some intervention.

As a result of influence from peers, movies, and other mass-media forces, many male teens feel they should be more "masculine." These males believe they need to be brave risk takers who should be the dominating and controlling figure in their male-female relationships. They

Table 3.3
Development of Independence

> Early (12–14 years)
> - less attention paid to parents
> - peer group begins to influence behavior and interests
> - struggle to forge an identity begins
>
> Middle (15–18 years)
> - your opinion of your parents declines, temporarily
> - much concern about your physical appearance
> - strong, influential relationships with peers
>
> Late (19–21 years)
> - increasing emotional stability
> - ability to be self-reliant
> - greater concern for others

are wrong. Often, adolescent girls like boys who are sensitive and look like Leonardo DiCaprio. Generally, girls want to be treated as equals. Some male teens find themselves torn between the two standards. Sadly, males may feel that they need to perform sexually in order to prove to their friends that they are manly. That is a mistake. You should strive to develop more emotional connections in your relationships rather than exclusively physical ties.

In order to sell their products, advertisers promote risky behaviors such as smoking and drinking. Some boys drink because they think everyone else is drinking, even though the belief that "everyone's doing it" is a myth. It is not uncommon for adolescents to drink because of peer pressure or to relieve pain or stress.

You do not need to participate in risky activities in order to be accepted by your peers. Research has shown that male teens may have a private self-image that's quite different from their public image. The private male may be friendly and loving; the more public male may take risks and/or be violent. How can you reconcile these two images?

A major part of your emotional development involves learning to resolve the conflicts between your private and public selves. You need to find a balance between being comfortable with your masculinity and maintaining positive relationships with females. And it is important that you learn to be sensible when faced with risky activities. It is not always easy to achieve these goals; some boys never do.

For many, it is useful to have a role model. Who is your hero? Though you might emulate a sports superstar, a coach, or an actor, research has shown that real heroes are more likely to be found among your parents, grandparents, older siblings, aunts, or uncles. Your hero should be some-

Table 3.4
Career Development

> Early (12–14 years)
> - concerned about the present
> - beginning to think in the abstract
>
> Middle (15–18 years)
> - increasingly goal oriented
> - intellectual concerns become more important
>
> Late (19–21 years)
> - future oriented
> - high level of intellectual thinking
> - serious concern about one's role in the world

one you respect and admire; you should model your behavior after that person. I also suggest that you try the following:

- spend time with your parent(s) doing fun activities
- talk to your parent(s) about things that bother you
- ask your parent(s) how they got through adolescence

While you may feel that your parents' adolescent struggles have no relevance in contemporary society, many of the issues that they faced at your age—and the ways they dealt with those issues—can help you today. It is okay for you to ask them about sensitive issues. I am sure they will appreciate your candor.

From your parents' perspective, it is also reasonable for them to do the following:

- engage you in discussion about some of the touchy issues of the adolescent years, including drugs, alcohol, sex, and emotions
- listen carefully and sensitively to what you are saying
- display their love for you
- make you comfortable and safe at home
- respect your privacy, especially your room, phone calls, and other communications
- be honest with you
- try to avoid nagging and preaching and being overly critical
- be willing to let you grow and develop emotionally during adolescence, letting you become an independent, decisive, critical thinking, and self-sufficient man by the end of adolescence

REFERENCES

Greydanus, Donald E., M.D., editor-in-chief. *Caring for Your Adolescent: Ages 12 to 21*. New York: Bantam Books, 1991.

McAnarney, Elizabeth, Richard Kreipe, Donald Orr, and George Comerci, editors. *Textbook of Adolescent Medicine*. Philadelphia: W. B. Saunders Co., 1992.

Pollack, William, M.D., *Real Boys*. New York: Random House, 1998.

Sanfilippo, Joseph S., M.D., Jordan W. Finkelstein, M.D., and Dennis M. Styne, M.D., editors. *Medical and Gynecologic Endocrinology, Adolescent Medicine: State of the Art Reviews*. Philadelphia: Hanley & Belfus, February 1994.

4

General Nutrition and Sports Nutrition

GENERAL NUTRITION

Females are not the only teens who are concerned with their appearance. Male teens focus on their bodies, especially their height and weight. And those who participate in sports are interested in the "competitive edge." This chapter will focus on general principles of nutrition for adolescent males and then review specific areas of nutrition that impact athletes.

In their race to leave for school or work, many adolescents skip breakfast. Sometimes, there is little or no time for lunch. When they do eat, it is frequently at fast food restaurants. So it is not surprising that the diet of many male teens does not meet even minimal nutritional requirements. Their intake of fruits, vegetables, and cereals may be low. And, with so many teens drinking juices, soft drinks, and beverages other than milk or other calcium-rich drinks, their consumption of calcium may be insufficient for a still-growing body.

From the pre-adolescent age of 10 to the postadolescent age of 20, the lean body mass of the average male increases by 75 pounds. In boys, this weight change is a result of growth in muscle mass, bones, and blood volume. Generally, at the peak of the male's growth spurt, he needs to store and utilize an extra 400 mg of calcium, 1.1 mg of iron, 0.50 mg of zinc, and 3800 mg of protein *every day*. These values are almost double those of an adolescent male who is not in the midst of a growth spurt. Calcium and protein are needed for bone and skeletal growth, iron is required for the synthesis of red blood cells. And without zinc, proper growth and sexual maturation will not take place.

The following values are the normal daily nutritional requirements for a male adolescent between the ages of 15 and 18, who weighs 145 pounds:

Calcium	1200 mg
Protein	59 grams
Iron	12 mg
Zinc	15 mg

Source: National Academy of Sciences, 1989.

Milk provides all four of these nutrients. An eight-ounce glass of milk has 300 mg of calcium, 8 grams of protein, 0.12 mg of iron, and 0.93 mg of zinc. Depending on the amount of fat in the milk you drink, an eight-ounce glass will have between 80 and 150 calories. Obviously, it would be wise to make milk one of the fluids that you include in your diet. For proper energy, the average adolescent male requires 41 calories per inch (of height) each day. So, if you are 70 inches tall, you need about 2,870 calories daily during your mid- to late adolescence.

Many of you have probably heard that you should take a vitamin to stay healthy. Is there any truth to that? If you are deficient in vitamins due to disease or poor diet, then supplementation is necessary. As an example, iron-deficiency anemia may occur in boys as they rapidly gain weight and grow. This is especially common if their diet is deficient in iron. Therefore, if you are anemic from low iron, then supplementation and dietary changes would be useful. The following are the recommended amounts of vitamins for boys between the ages of 15 and 18:

Vitamin A	1000 ug
Vitamin B6	2 mg
Vitamin B12	2 mg
Vitamin C	60 mg
Vitamin D	10 ug
Vitamin E	10 mg
Vitamin K	65 ug
Folate	200 ug
Niacin	20 mg
Riboflavin	18 mg
Thiamine	15 mg

Source: National Academy of Sciences, 1989.

Most well-balanced diets contain these amounts of vitamins. Do you run the risk of problems if you consume too few or too many vitamins? Yes. See the following chart of some potential problems. Unless you have a vitamin deficiency, you should not assume that more is better.

Vitamin	Deficiency	Excess
A	night blindness	loss of hair
B1	neurological problems	unknown
B6	depression, skin problems	sensitivity to sun
B12	anemia	unknown
C	bleeding gums	kidney stones
D	rickets	kidney calcium
E	unclear	bleeding
K	bleeding (rare)	probably none

Unless it is carefully balanced, a vegetarian diet may give rise to deficiencies. When the diet is strictly vegetarian, with no animal products, it is called *vegan*. If it includes milk, it is called *lacto-vegetarian*; if it includes milk and eggs, it is *lacto-ovo vegetarian*. During adolescence, it is particularly important for you to obtain adequate amounts of protein, B12, calcium, and iron. B12 is found only in animal products. So a vegan may be at risk for B12 deficiency and might wish to supplement his diet. Milk will supply calcium, B12, and protein; iron is found in enriched cereal and leafy green vegetables.

During adolescence, protein usually supplies about 12 percent to 14 percent of energy. But, generally, the energy supplied by protein is not utilized during sports. Males between the ages of 15 and 18 need about 0.40 gram of protein per pound of weight. Thus, if you weigh 150 pounds, you require 60 grams of protein each day. In a national survey, it was determined that the average daily protein intake for males was 107 grams per day—well above the recommended amount. Therefore, if you are an adolescent male living in the United States, it is highly unlikely that you are protein deficient.

There is some disagreement among professionals about how much fat should be included in the male adolescent's diet. Most authorities believe that a fat intake of more than 40 percent of the total daily calories is too much. In fact, some believe that the limit should be set at 30 percent or lower. According to national data, the average male adolescent consumes a diet of about 37 percent fat. While there are four calories in a gram of protein or carbohydrates, each gram of fat has nine calories. So it is relatively easy to become overweight from a diet with too much fat.

Fat may be utilized as an energy source during exercise. And, over time, training increases the likelihood that more fat will be used as energy during exercise.

Carbohydrates are a major source of energy for the body. They are a source of quick and short-term energy.

No more than 50 percent of your daily calories should come from carbohydrates. Unfortunately, according to surveys, more than 25 percent of the total carbohydrates in the diet of most male teens is provided by table sugar or high fructose corn syrup. A 1997 Centers for Disease Control and Prevention survey found that two-thirds of male adolescents ate less than five servings of fruits and vegetables daily.

The following is a table of the daily dietary guidelines that male teens should follow.

Bread, cereal, rice, pasta	6 to 11 servings (Serving = 1 slice of bread, ½ cup of cooked rice, pasta, or cereal, 4–5 crackers, or 10 ounces of ready-to-eat cereal)
Vegetables	3 to 5 servings (Serving = ½ cup of chopped raw or cooked vegetables or 1 cup of leafy raw vegetable)
Fruits	2 to 4 servings (Serving = 1 apple, ¾ cup of juice, ½ cup of canned fruit, or ¼ cup of dried fruit)
Milk, yogurt, cheese	2 to 3 servings (Serving = 1 cup of milk or yogurt or 1 ½–2 ounces of cheese)
Meat, poultry, fish, beans, eggs, nuts	2 to 3 servings (Serving = 3 ounces of lean meat, fish, or poultry; 1 ounce meat = ½ cup of cooked beans, 1 egg, and 2 tablespoons of peanut butter)
Fats, oils, and sweets	Eat sparingly

Here's a sample healthy meal plan for one day.

Breakfast
Bowl of cereal
Glass of milk
2 slices of toast or bagel with jam
Lunch
Sandwich (meat/fish/protein source)
Milk
Fruit

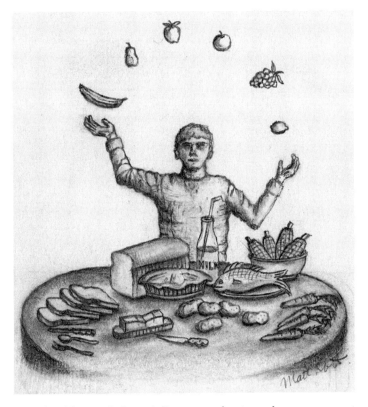

You should eat a balanced diet every day to make sure you get the right amounts of food from the different food groups.

Vegetable

Snack

Juice

Fruit

Dinner

Poultry/Meat/Fish/Pasta

Two vegetables

Bread/roll

Milk

Dessert

Snack

Fruit

FAST FOOD

Though most people associate fast food restaurants with foods that are higher in fat and sodium (salt), it is possible to eat at fast food restaurants and have a relatively nutritious, lower-calorie meal. Let's look at two different meals.

Food	Calories	Fat (gms/serving)	Sodium (mg)
Quarter pounder w/cheese	530	30	1,310
Large french fries	540	26	350
Shake (8oz.)	360	9	250
Total	1,430	65	1,910

Source: McDonald's Corporation Web site, January 24, 2000.

For those who wish to maintain a healthier diet, this meal has problems. Since the daily caloric intake for adolescent males is just under 3,000, this typical fast food meal comprises a large chunk of the day's calories—around 48 percent. And it has a lot of fat. In order to keep your daily fat consumption to approximately 30 percent of your diet, you should consume about 900 calories of fat. In the meal specified above, grams are from fat, and each of these grams has nine calories. This meal has 585 calories from fat—65 percent of the daily fat requirement.

There is also a problem with sodium. Eighteen-year-old males need about 500 mg of sodium per day. Excessive sodium has no positive health benefit and may lead to elevated blood pressure. This meal has far too much sodium and too little calcium.

While an occasional meal like this probably is okay for most teens, those who regularly eat this type food may face negative health consequences. Let's look at a healthier fast food meal:

Food	Calories	Fat (gms/serving)	Sodium (mg)
Grilled chicken sandwich	440	20	1,040
Salad with ranch dressing	265	21	550
Low-fat milk	100	25	115
Total	805	43.5	1,705

Source: McDonald's Corporation Web site, January 24, 2000.

Though far from ideal, this is a better alternative. Yet, it also contains a lot of fat and sodium for one meal. So even the better fast food choices may pose problems. If you frequently eat at fast food restaurants, take

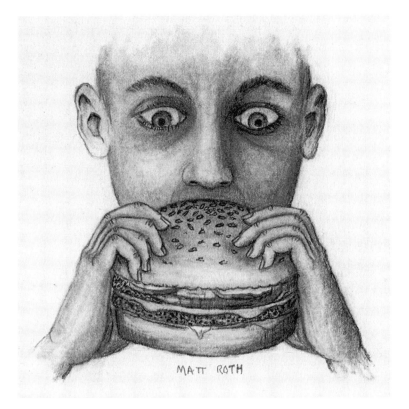

Fast foods may have excessive amounts of calories, fat, and sodium.

the time to read the nutritional information of the different offerings and try to select the most healthful choices.

NUTRITION AND GROWTH

Will eating extra calories boost your growth? Eating sufficient calories will enable you to grow as tall as your genes have been programmed for you to grow. Excess calories will not make you grow any taller, and they may make you fat, even obese. There are several formulas to determine your ultimate height. These are approximate; some individuals grow taller and others shorter than the formulas predicted.

Formula #1: Take your father's height. Add five inches. Add your mother's height. Then divide by 2. This should be your ultimate height. For example, if your father is 70 inches tall and your mother is 65 inches, the calculation is as follows.

$$(70 + 5) + 65 = 140 \div 2 = 70 \text{ inches}$$

Formula #2: Ask your parents for your early childhood growth chart. Then look to see how tall you were at the age of two. Double that figure.

Formula #3: Add your father's and mother's heights together. Divide the figure you get by 2. Then add four inches. If your parents are either on the tall or short side, this formula may have an error of at least one inch. So, if your parents' average height is 67.5 inches, you add four inches and have your ultimate height of 71.5 inches. This is close to but not the same as the first formula.

Remember that while these formulas are estimates for height, they may have serious limitations. According to the first formula, my son, Brett, who is now in his mid-20s, should be about 5-foot-8½-inches tall. The second formula places him at 6 feet. He is actually 6-foot-2.

What is a good weight for your height? Here is a formula that provides a rough estimate. You begin with 106 pounds for your first 60 inches. Then you add six pounds for each additional inch of height. Thus, if you are 16 years old and 68 inches tall, your weight should be about 154 pounds (106 pounds + 8 × 6). Refer to the Boy's 2 to 18 Years growth chart (Figure 3.1) published by the Centers for Disease Control. At age 16, a boy who is 68 inches is in the 45th percentile. Find the 45th percentile on the weight growth chart for a 16-year-old. That will tell you what a good approximate weight would be for your height. The growth chart I use says that a 16-year-old male teen who is 68 inches tall should weight 135 pounds. Again, the formulas do not agree. But they do provide an acceptable range. And, each person is different. You should expect variation. Some boys have larger frames and bigger bones, with bigger and heavier muscles. Others are thinner and have less muscle.

The Body Mass Index (BMI) formula serves as a relatively easy way to determine if your weight is about what it should be. Before calculating your BMI, you must determine your weight in kilograms (pounds divided by 2.2) and your height in meters (inches divided by 39.4). After you have those figures, you may begin by squaring (multiplying by itself) your height in meters. Then divide your weight in kilograms by your squared height. For example, let's say you weigh 170 pounds. Begin by dividing 170 by 2.2. That gives us 77.3 kilograms. And let's say you are 70 inches tall. When 70 is divided by 39.4, you have 1.78 meters. Now, square your height in meters (1.78 times 1.78). That gives us 3.17. And divide your weight in kilograms (77.3) by 3.17. From this, you have 24.4. For male adolescents between 15 and 18, a value of 30 or more indicates obesity and 25–29 means overweight. Values between 18 and 24 represent the appropriate weight. A value of less than 18 could mean that you are underweight. Because of their extra muscle mass, this formula does not work well for body builders, and it is best utilized for adolescents who are older and have completed their growth. See table 4.1 for calculated Body Mass Index values.

WEIGHT ISSUES

Adolescent males are also concerned with their weight. As previously noted, there are methods to determine if your weight is generally appropriate for your height. No method is perfect. The growth charts are only valid for people 18 years of age and younger. Insurance company charts tend to be for adults rather than teens, and those formulas fail to factor in body frame. Obviously, people who are big boned and broad shouldered should carry more weight. The BMI is a more accurate method to determine if someone is overweight. Skin-fold measurements are also good for detecting percentage of body fat.

About 15–20 percent of adolescents are overweight. For our purposes, overweight may be defined as 20 percent above the ideal weight for your height. So the teen who has an average build, and is 70 inches tall, has an ideal weight of 166 pounds. That teen would be termed overweight if he weighed 200 pounds. The stricter BMI would term him overweight at 175 pounds. Morbid obesity is defined as weighing 100 pounds above your ideal.

In general, most male adolescents are not overweight as a result of illness. While, in some cases, adolescents gain weight from problems with hormones, such as thyroid or cortisol, the vast majority of overweight problems are caused by teens who take in more energy, in the form of calories, than they use. Unless a teen gets sufficient exercise, excess calories are usually stored as fat cells. With exercise, the excess calories may be stored as muscle. There are also teens who have a genetic propensity to be overweight. And some environmental factors—such as the types of food in your home, your ethnic background, the number of members of your nuclear family, how much television you watch, and whether you live in the city or a rural area—predispose you to weight problems.

Of course, everybody knows thin people who are able to eat huge amounts of food without putting on an ounce. But, most people gain weight when they eat too much. Let's put this into perspective. For every extra 3,000 calories you eat—above what your body needs to function— you will gain one pound. Remember the McDonald's large fries. Well, one order had 450 calories. It would take about a five-mile run to burn that amount of calories. Or you could cut something else from your diet. If you don't plan to exercise, it might be easier just to skip the fries.

Teens who are overweight from excessive caloric intake know that losing weight is not easy. Nevertheless, to protect their present and fu-

Table 4.1
Body Mass Index

Weight (pounds)	Height (inches)																
	60	61	62	63	64	65	66	67	68	69	70	71	72	73	74	75	76
130	25	25	24	23	22	22	21	20	20	19	19	18	18	17	17	16	16
135	26	26	25	24	23	22	22	21	21	20	19	19	18	18	17	17	16
140	27	26	26	25	24	23	23	22	21	21	20	20	19	18	18	17	17
145	28	27	27	26	25	24	23	23	22	21	21	20	20	19	19	18	18
150	29	28	27	27	26	25	24	23	23	22	22	21	20	20	19	19	18
155	30	29	28	27	27	26	25	24	24	23	22	22	21	20	20	19	19
160	31	30	29	28	27	27	26	25	24	24	23	22	22	21	21	20	19
165	32	31	30	29	28	27	27	26	25	24	24	23	22	22	21	21	20
170	33	32	31	30	29	28	27	27	26	25	24	24	23	22	22	21	21
175	34	33	32	31	30	29	28	27	27	26	25	24	24	23	22	22	21
180	35	34	33	32	31	30	29	28	27	27	26	25	24	24	23	22	22
185	36	35	34	33	32	31	30	29	28	27	27	26	25	24	24	23	23
190	37	36	35	34	33	32	31	30	29	28	27	26	26	25	24	24	23
195	38	37	36	35	33	32	31	31	30	29	28	27	26	25	25	24	24
200	39	38	37	35	34	33	32	31	30	30	29	28	27	26	26	25	24
205	40	39	37	36	35	34	33	32	31	30	29	29	28	27	26	26	25
210	41	40	38	37	36	35	34	33	32	31	30	29	28	28	27	26	26

A BMI of 30 or more indicates obesity.
A BMI of 25–29 indicates overweight.
A BMI of 18–24 is appropriate.
A BMI of less than 18 indicates underweight.

ture health, they should make changes in their behavior. If you are such a teen, you should moderate your daily caloric intake, increase the amount of exercise you do, and ask for support from family members and friends. In general, eat about 50 percent of the normally required calories (about 1,450 calories) in a balanced diet that includes lots of fruits and vegetables.

Most adolescent males refuse to attend weight-loss support programs. While such programs have helped countless people, it is possible to lose weight without such a structure. But you need to be highly motivated.

I had a 15-year-old patient who was about 30 pounds overweight; he was 60 inches tall and weighed 140 pounds. He was unhappy with his appearance, and his ability to compete on the playing field was diminished. Moreover, none of his clothes fit. I suggested that he modify his diet, cut his caloric intake, and find fun ways to exercise daily. Slowly, his weight dropped. At his last check-up, he was 63 inches tall and weighed 115 pounds. He showed a renewed sense of confidence and self-esteem, and he is thrilled with his thinner appearance. Like my patient, you can lose your excess weight. But it does take determination and family support.

Adolescent males who are 20 percent or more below their ideal weight are termed underweight. Underweight males rarely have the problems that come with excess weight, such as high blood fats and increased blood pressure. But underweight males may have problems with their thyroid or other hormones. Your medical provider can determine if you require testing. And underweight teens may underachieve athletically. They may also have underlying medical problems.

For example, I had a 16-year-old male patient who began to lose weight, even though he was eating quite well and craving sugar. Curiously, he also was urinating frequently and often had to get up at night to go to the bathroom. When he came in for an office visit, he reported that a marked loss of energy had forced him to discontinue his participation in after-school sports. It did not take me long to determine that he had developed diabetes. Thankfully, he responded well to treatment. My patient now checks his sugar levels several times each day and self-administers the appropriate levels of insulin. He had regained his weight and has returned to competitive sports.

This example illustrates the importance of monitoring how you feel as well as your weight. If you note that you are losing weight without trying to lose weight, you should consult your medical provider. Also, if you gain excessive amounts of weight, you could have a hormonal problem. Additionally, any major change in your energy levels—whether you have too little energy or too much—may be a signal for you to seek medical attention.

While eating disorders such as anorexia nervosa are fairly common among female teens, they are rare among males. Still, male teens and their parents should be aware that they do occur. And, as with overweight teens, teens who have parents who were thin adolescents may have a tendency to be thin—at least during their teens. As a teen I could eat anything. And since information on proper nutrition was essentially nonexistent in the 1950s and 1960s, my mother would buy me extraheavy cream, which I would drink in tall glasses. Needless to say, those days are long gone.

A new disorder that causes distress and impaired social interactions in male teens has recently been observed. Called *muscle dysmorphia*, this disorder involves preoccupation with the size of one's muscles. Even though he might appear to be very muscular, a male teen with this disorder feels that his muscular development is insufficient and inadequate. In order to build muscle mass, some people with this significant disorder of body image abuse anabolic steroids. Some also take countless amounts of supplements in order to increase the bulk of their muscles. Since they are preoccupied with and ashamed of their body appearance, teens with muscle dysmorphia are afraid to take off their shirt, which interferes with their everyday functioning. Treatments are available from qualified professions.

Some boys define masculinity in terms of physical strength and toughness, and a need for respect from peers and girlfriends. They are reluctant to talk about emotional issues. Researchers define these boys as having a "masculine ideology." Boys with this view of masculinity are at a higher risk for substance abuse, educational problems, risky sexual behaviors, and problems with the law.

SPORTS NUTRITION

If you are an athlete, you probably already know that your performance is affected by what you eat and drink or fail to eat and drink. But you might not know some of the subtle ways to increase your competitive edge.

While you were still in early puberty, exercise and diet had little effect on the size and strength of your muscles. The relatively low level of androgenic hormones, the substances that stimulate the development of masculine traits, prevented the formation of significant muscle mass. However, as puberty draws to a close, the levels of these hormones begin to rise, and exercise and proper nutrition increase the size and strength of muscles.

So what is the relationship between exercise and the three basic sources of energy—carbohydrates, protein, and fats? The average 154-pound non-overweight male has lots of energy stored in his body in the following way:

Carbohydrates	1,840 calories
Protein	40,000 calories
Fat	140,000 calories

That is sufficient energy to run for 11.8 days straight without stopping to eat—an incredible feat! If you could run a six-minute mile for this amount of time, you would have enough fuel in your body to run from Boston to San Francisco and still have some fuel left to go on to Berkeley.

Carbohydrates are present as the sugar glucose in the blood or stored as glycogen in the muscles and liver. For a short burst of energy, such as a 100-yard sprint, your body will burn glucose. If your body requires more sustained energy, as in a marathon, it will use muscle or liver glycogen. We often hear about marathoners who eat carbohydrates, such as pasta, before a race. Eating excess carbohydrates for several days before a race allows the body to build up glycogen in the muscles and liver. On the day prior to the event, athletes try to get more rest, "load up on carbs," and increase their intake of fluids. Theoretically, this regimen allows for greater endurance during the race.

Generally, protein is not metabolized during athletics. It is only when the athletic event requires a longer, sustained energy flow—such as in a marathon—that protein may be burned. Most marathoners simply increase their caloric load to compensate for their caloric loss thereby maintaining protein balance. Even though there may be some destruction of protein from the wear and tear on the body, there is no need to increase dietary protein.

Many teens erroneously believe that weight training increases the body's need for protein. As we noted earlier in the chapter, the current recommendation for protein is approximately 0.40 gram per pound of your weight. Weight lifters may need a little more—0.60 to 0.75 grams of protein per pound. Because Americans already eat a diet that is high in protein, there is usually no reason to increase your daily protein intake. So, if you weigh 150 pounds and you are a weight lifter, your protein intake should be no more than 113 grams.

What are the protein values of some common foods? The following list may provide an introduction.

Food	Grams of Protein
1 cup skim milk	8
3 oz. chicken, fish, or meat	21
1 large egg	7
1 oz cheddar cheese	8
2 tbs. peanut butter	9

Source: The Yale Guide to Children's Nutrition, 1996.

Clearly, a healthy adolescent male can reach his daily protein requirement without much difficulty. Protein supplements are unnecessary. In
fact, too much protein can lead to dehydration and kidney problems.
There is little scientific evidence that consumption of large quantities of
protein supplements will enhance performance, increase muscle mass, or
bolster strength.

One of my patients was a 19-year-old body builder who wanted to
become a police officer. Believing he was in excellent health, he took the
physical exam and the required laboratory tests. Blood tests determined
that his kidney function was abnormal. At this point, he admitted taking
protein supplements. Additional blood tests found that he was suffering
from mild kidney failure. Fortunately, once he discontinued the protein
supplements, his kidney function improved, and he continued to do
body building without protein supplementation.

Fat is a tremendous source of energy. One pound of fat (454 grams)
can supply enough energy (4,086 calories) for a marathoner to run 30
miles. Training may allow the body to utilize fat in lieu of carbohydrates, at least temporarily. That is why people who have high blood
cholesterol levels are asked to exercise. Cholesterol is a fatty substance
that is necessary for some body functions such as production of hormones, but in excessive levels it can be deposited in the arteries and
lead to heart disease. Moderate exercise may help reduce the harmful
LDL cholesterol and produce more HDL cholesterol, which protects
against heart disease. In any case, it is important for all of us to follow
a diet that is low in saturated fats such as butter, marbleized meats, and
cream and higher in unsaturated fats such as those found in olive oil
and nuts. There is a direct relationship between the amount of saturated
fat in your diet and your cholesterol level. Unsaturated fats are classified as monounsaturated or polyunsaturated. Monounsaturated fats are
found in olive oil and may reduce your LDL cholesterol. Polyunsaturated fats found in fish or corn oil have a more profound effect on lowering LDL cholesterol.

Do extra vitamins and minerals improve your athletic performance?
Usually not. However, if you have an underlying illness, such as iron-
deficiency anemia, then your athletic performance could be compromised by the insufficient quantity of iron in your system. In this case,
iron supplementation would be indicated. But, since the vast majority of
male adolescents do not suffer from iron deficiency, they usually have
adequate stores of iron.

Will gaining weight make you more competitive? If you are under-
weight for your height, you should exercise and consume more calories.
Exercising will convert your excess calories into muscle, rather than fat.
Although many believe that exercise must be rigorous to be effective,

that is not true. A daily exercise program is probably best for adolescent males. This could include brisk walking for 30 minutes, jogging for 15 minutes, or a 15-minute session of basketball. Besides building muscles, exercise reduces fat, stress, and weight, and promotes your psychological well-being. To gain weight you may wish to eat between meals, eat higher-calorie, low-bulk foods, such as lasagna, or even drink a commercially prepared supplement for weight gain. Sports bars may also help with weight gain. A Clif bar has 250 calories, including 8 grams of protein. A PowerBar has 230 calories, 45 grams of carbohydrates, 2.5 grams of fat, and 10 grams of protein.

Sometimes, male teens, who participate in certain sports, such as wrestling, feel that they need to be in a lower weight class. To reduce their weight, teens may attempt "self-induced dehydration." For several reasons, this is a very bad idea. Dehydration is not good for your overall health. Moreover, studies have shown that high school wrestlers who "made weight" had a decline in grip strength and decreased levels of energy. "Making weight" could impair your performance. And keep in mind that in their attempts to "make weight," several college wrestlers have died.

What is the best type of meal to eat before an athletic competition? Try to have a high-carbohydrate, low-protein, low-fat meal. Too much protein may lead to dehydration, and too much fat will impede the transit of food from the stomach to the small intestine. And your meal should also include lots of fluids. Carbohydrates pass through the stomach quickly, so that part of digestion will not be an issue during the event. But do try to eat several hours before the event begins. Some people feel that if they eat a sports bar just prior to the event, they will have a competitive edge. It is unclear whether that is true.

Here are a couple of sample meals to eat prior to competition:

Meal #1

Pasta

Juice

Bread

Fruit

Meal #2

Cereal with low-fat milk

Low-fat yogurt

Bagel

Vegetable juice

Fruit

We all hear a great deal about nutritional ergogenics or nutritional substances that are said to improve athletic performance. These include creatine, amino acids, chromium, carnitine, caffeine, DHEA, and androstenedione. There are no definitive statistics on the numbers of males between the ages of 15 and 18 who use nutritional supplements. However, up to 13 percent of all college athletes have used creatine and 8 percent have used amino acids.

Creatine is a natural substance that is produced by the liver, kidneys, and pancreas. It has also been available commercially since 1993. Cells with high-energy requirements use phosphocreatine, which is derived from creatine, to generate energy; there is enough of this substance in your body for 10 seconds of high-intensity activity. In a review of 31 studies of repetitive high-energy and short-duration tasks (such as weight lifting), it was found that taking creatine by mouth may modestly improve performance. While users of creatine tend to gain weight, this may be the result of water retention in the tissues as well as protein synthesis. It is possible that creatine users are more prone to muscle strain; there are also reports of muscle cramping, rashes, vomiting, diarrhea, anxiety, fatigue, and nervousness from creatine usage. No studies have been conducted on the long-term effects of creatine on the body. Creatine is not cheap. A daily dose is about $3. Its use is not banned by the International Olympic Committee or the National Collegiate Athletic Association.

To raise their daily protein intake, athletes may take amino acid supplementation. Amino acids are basic building blocks of all proteins. Some believe that excess protein from amino acids may help repair their bodies after strenuous exercise. Others feel that the ingestion of certain amino acids will increase the production of creatine or growth hormone. In fact, as has been noted, American males consume more protein than they need. Do you still believe that you need more protein? Before taking supplementation, try this simple method. Calculate your daily protein intake for one week. If you are a gymnast or wrestler, you may be on weight restriction, and it is possible that you are not getting sufficient protein. Although it has previously been noted that a non-athletic male needs around 0.40 gram of protein per pound, this could be doubled for participants in certain sports, such as body building. Evaporated milk, egg whites, and soy powder are relatively inexpensive sources of protein.

Chromium, a trace element found in foods such as mushrooms, prunes, nuts, and asparagus, is an aid in the metabolism of glucose, fat, and protein. It helps insulin, a hormone necessary for the regulation of blood sugar, bind to tissue and enhance its performance. At present, there is no accurate way to determine chromium deficiency.

Many athletes believe that chromium increases muscle mass and decreases fat in the body. This notion is based on the fact that when insulin is low or ineffective, less protein and sugar and more fat enter cells. If chromium does play a role in the binding of insulin to cells, then it should make insulin more effective. In one study that failed to prove that football players benefited from chromium supplementation, chromium was given to players over a nine-week period. Their body composition and strength at the end of the nine weeks was no different from the players who did not receive chromium. Thus, current, research neither supports nor refutes the benefits of chromium for athletes.

Carnitine is synthesized in the body from the amino acids lysine and methionine. It is also important in the metabolism of certain fatty acids that may yield energy during high-intensity sports. Theoretically, carnitine should be useful in endurance sports. But research into its effects on athletic performance is inconclusive. The daily cost of carnitine supplementation is approximately $2.60.

It appears that caffeine enhances endurance. Caffeine is found in coffee, tea, colas, chocolates, and other foods; it is also available in over-the-counter form. There are many side effects from caffeine, including nervousness, wakefulness, upset stomach, and increased heart rate, urination, and blood pressure. Individuals become dependent on caffeine and have withdrawal symptoms, including headache and fatigue, when they stop taking it. Many adolescents avoid caffeine because of these problems. Caffeine is banned by the International Olympic Committee.

Regrettably, in an attempt to improve performance, some adolescents turn to androgenic steroids and speed, described in Chapter 6. These substances are illegal and potentially dangerous.

In the body, DHEA (dehydroepiandrosterone), which is produced by the adrenal glands, is converted to testosterone and estrogen (female hormone). The adrenal glands, located on the kidneys, manufacture hormones critical to metabolic and reproductive functions. No studies have demonstrated that DHEA increases muscle mass and strength in young athletes. At certain intake levels, males taking DHEA may develop breasts, and such growth may be permanent.

Androstenedione is a hormone manufactured by the adrenal gland and the testicles. Eventually, it is converted to a female hormone (estrone) and testosterone. Some athletes believe that it increases muscle mass, and, in so doing, heightens performance. There is no scientific basis for this belief. On the contrary, if you have too much testosterone in your system from self-administered androstenedione, you may become virilized. What does it mean to be virilized? You may grow hair on your back and experience the premature onset of baldness. Your growth may be halted—even if you are still growing you may develop acne. If you already have acne, it may get worse. Your testicles may shrink, and your sperm count may drop. Some of your bodily testosterone is converted to female hormones. So if you raise your testosterone levels by taking androstenedione, you may actually be raising the levels of female hormones in your body. As a result, some individuals taking this hormone have developed breast tissue. Androstenedione should be avoided.

Everyone knows that medical problems may develop during sports events. (Sports injuries are discussed in detail in Chapter 7.) During a hot and humid summer day, one of my patients, who was 17 years old, developed severe leg cramps at the end of a soccer practice. Rushed to the hospital, physicians determined that he was severely dehydrated. He began to urinate only after receiving five quarts of intravenous fluids. In retrospect, he said that because he did not feel thirsty, he did not drink sufficient fluids during practice. As a result, he suffered from heat cramps, which are painful, and sustained muscle contractions, usually of the lower leg muscles.

How much water should you drink during exercise? The easiest and best way to determine how much water to drink is to monitor your weight before and after workouts. If you lose a pound from your workout, you should drink 16 ounces of water. In other words, replace the weight you lose with the same amount of fluids. During an athletic event, periodically drink cold water, even if you are not thirsty. If you depend solely on your level of thirst, half of your sweat losses may not be replaced, so drink more than you need.

If you become dehydrated during exercise, you may exhibit a number of symptoms. These should be a red flag. Stop immediately and drink some fluids. You may have a decreased urine output and an elevated heart rate due to loss of fluid volume in your blood stream. Your mental acuity, strength, and stamina may also be diminished. Why? Because there has been some reduction in the volume of blood that is pumped with each heartbeat so your brain, muscles, and kidneys are not receiving an optimal blood supply for proper functioning.

Perspiration during exercise is the body's way of dissipating excess heat. When you perspire, you lose fluids and salts such as sodium and chloride. To optimize your performance, you should match the fluid and electrolyte loss by drinking adequate amounts of fluid that contain a little sugar. Because cold fluids transit the stomach faster than warm or hot fluids, cold drinks are a better choice. Cold fluids also stimulate your thirst mechanism and counteract the heat you are producing from exercise.

Inadequate fluid replacement may lead to heat exhaustion or heat stroke. Your body's thermoregulatory mechanism may become impaired, leading to a higher body temperature. Heat exhaustion may occur when dehydration exceeds 3 percent of your body's weight. Thus, if you weigh 150 pounds and have lost five pounds from perspiration, you risk dehydration. Athletes with heat exhaustion may experience weakness, dizziness, fainting, and nausea. Heat stroke is more serious and may be life threatening. During heat stroke, the athlete is in shock. Treatment includes hydration and lowering of the body's temperature. While immediate medical care is important for heat exhaustion, in the case of heat stroke, medical care is urgent and must not be delayed.

REFERENCES

Clancy, S. P., P. K. Clarkson, M. S. DeCheke, K. Nosaka, P. S. Freedson, J. J. Cunningham, and B. Valentine. "Effects of Chromium Picolinate Supplementation on Body Composition, Strength, and Urinary Chromium Loss in Football Players." *International Journal of Sports Nutrition* 4 (June 1994) 2: 142–153.

Dyment, Paul G., editor. *Sports Medicine: Health Care for Young Athletes.* 2nd Edition. Elk Grove Village, Ill.: American Academy of Pediatrics, 1991.

Greydanus, Donald E., Dilip R. Patel, and Eugene F. Luckstead, editors. *Office Orthopedics and Sports Medicine, Adolescent Medicine: State of the Arts Review.* Philadelphia: Hanley & Belfus, October 1998.

Hall, S. S. "The Bully in the Mirror." *New York Times Magazine* (August 22, 1999): 30–65.

Hergenroeder, Albert C., James G. Garrick. *Sports Medicine: The Pediatric Clinics of North America.* Philadelphia: W. B. Saunders Company, October 1990.

Juhn, M. S. "Oral Creatine Supplementation." *The Physician and Sportsmedicine* 27 (May 1999) 5:47–56.

Kleinman, Ronald E., editor. *Pediatric Nutrition Handbook, Fourth Edition.* Elk Grove Village, Ill.: American Academy of Pediatrics, 1998.

National Academy of Sciences. "Recommended Dietary Allowances." 10th Edition. Washington, D.C.: National Academy Press, 1989.

Nussbaum, Michael P., and Johanna T. Dwyer, editors. *Adolescent Nutrition and Eating Disorders, Adolescent Medicine: State of the Art Reviews.* Philadelphia: Henley & Belfus, October 1992.

Pope, H. G., A. J. Gruber, P. Choi, and K. A. Phillips. "Muscle Dysmorphia. An Underrecognized Form of Body Dysmorphic Disorder." *Psychosmatics* 38 (1997) 6: 549–557.

Strasburger, Victor C., and Robert T. Brown. *Adolescent Medicine: A Practical Guide.* Boston: Little, Brown and Co., 1991.

Tamborlane, William V., editor. *The Yale Guide to Children's Nutrition.* New Haven, Conn.: Yale University Press, 1996.

5

Sexuality

It is a reality many adults prefer to ignore. Large numbers of teens are sexually active. Just listen to the findings of a 1998 national survey from the Centers for Disease Control. Forty-nine percent of high school males reported that they had had sexual intercourse at least once. Of these, 9.4 percent had sexual intercourse prior to age 13. Eighteen percent had already had four or more partners. And 33 percent were currently sexually active.

But there were even more startling statistics. The survey determined that only 63 percent of the males used condoms during their last act of sexual intercourse. In an age when unprotected sex may lead to sexually transmitted disease, permanent illness, or even death, almost half the teens surveyed had unprotected sex. Thirty-one percent of the teens admitted that sexual intercourse was accompanied by the use of drugs and/or alcohol, and 5 percent of the males noted that they had impregnated a partner.

In his 1984 nationwide study of teen sexual acts, Robert Coles, M.D., a Harvard psychiatrist, found that even without sexual intercourse, large numbers of teens are sexually active. Forty percent of 17–18-year-old girls reported performing oral sex on males (fellatio) and 33 percent of boys the same age reported performing oral sex on females (cunnilingus).

Clearly, it is important that all teens have greater awareness of sexuality issues. Burying one's head in the sand is not a solution. Knowledge and education are vital. As a result, this chapter will include an overview of birth control, sexually transmitted diseases, acquaintance rape, sexual abuse, and concerns relevant to gay teens.

From my experience, males are now using condoms far more fre-

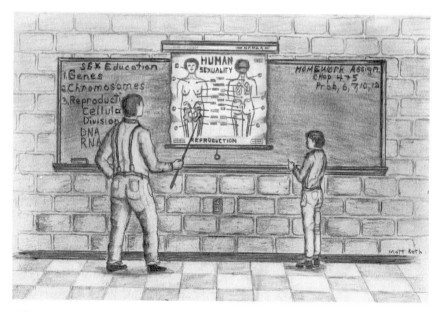

It is important for all teens to have a solid awareness of sexuality issues. Knowledge and education are vital.

quently than they did 15 years ago. But all too many still come up with numerous excuses for not using them. I hear the same reasons over and over again—"Condoms were not available" or "She wouldn't get pregnant from one sexual episode" or "She says it decreases the sensation."

Among female teens, birth control pills are the most popular method of contraception. Diaphragms, intrauterine devices, or long-acting hormone injections are far less common. At present, teenage males have three contraceptive choices.

Abstinence. Although you can contract sexually transmitted diseases from other types of sexual activities, abstaining from sexual intercourse is an excellent way to guard against pregnancy.

Withdrawal. While withdrawal is a method of contraception, I never recommend it. First of all, even prior to climax, sperm may be released in pre-ejaculate. So it is possible to get your partner pregnant using this method. Second, it is quite difficult to properly time the withdrawal. You may be as careful as possible and seminal fluid may spill. The failure rate for withdrawal is around 19 percent. For those who are perfectly fastidious, the failure rate is 4 percent. But withdrawal has another important downside. It does not protect you or your partner from any of the sexually transmitted diseases.

Condoms. Much has been written about condoms, and, regrettably, they are the subject of countless jokes. It is important to know what they can

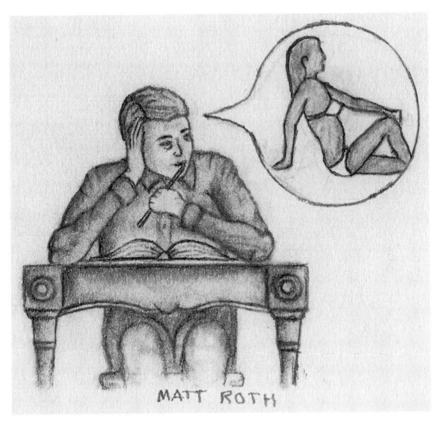

It is normal for male teens to daydream about sexual themes.

and cannot do. Condoms do not provide absolute protection against pregnancy. And they are only as good as how they are put on and when they are taken off. Although the failure rate is typically about 12 percent, it may be as high as 33 percent. With absolutely perfect use, the failure rate diminishes to 3 percent. Condoms used with a spermicide have a failure rate of up to 5 percent. However, with perfect use, it is typically less than that.

Hint: Always use a condom containing a spermicide such as nonoxynol 9.

Condoms are made from one of two kinds of materials—natural lambskin or latex. Some people contend that lambskin increases sensation. I am not sure that is true. Moreover, lambskin is more expensive than latex, and there is at least a theoretical risk that some viruses can be transmitted through the lambskin pores. Latex condoms are a better choice. They come in a variety of types. Ribbed, textured, and lubricated

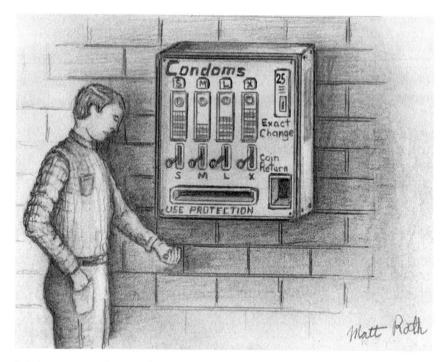

It is important to know what condoms can and cannot do. For example, they do not provide absolute protection against pregnancy.

condoms reduce sensation less than other types of condoms. Even if condoms do reduce sexual sensations, they tend to promote the length of intercourse. Note that condoms, which are all manufacturer tested, have an expiration date on the package. Do not use a condom after its expiration date. And do not store condoms in your wallet. The pressure may cause tiny tears, which would reduce their effectiveness. *Never* attempt to reuse a condom, which could easily split. After one use, a condom should be carefully discarded.

Important Point: If a condom splits or falls off, and there is leakage of seminal fluid into or around your partner's genitals, make sure she sees a medical provider so that emergency contraception—the morning after pill—may be prescribed.

You do not have to be 18 or 21 to purchase condoms. They have no age restriction, so feel free to purchase condoms at your local drugstore. Not that long ago, you had to ask for condoms at the counter. Fortunately, most are now displayed in the aisles. Also, some restaurants have condom-dispensing machines in their restrooms. Condoms are quite portable, and, at about 50 cents each, relatively inexpensive. Perhaps the only negative aspects to condoms are that they may briefly disrupt sex, and some people are allergic to latex.

What is the correct way to put on a condom?

1. When opening the package, be careful not to rip the condom.
2. Before putting on the condom, the penis must be erect. Either partner should place the condom on the penis prior to genital or anal contact.
3. Place the rolled rim against the head of the penis and unroll it down to the base of the penis. If it does not unroll, then it is inside out. Start with a new condom and roll correctly toward the base of the penis. Leave about one-half inch of space at the tip of the condom to hold the seminal fluid.
4. Some condoms are lubricated. If you are using one that is not lubricated, use a natural or artificial lubricant, such as water or K-Y jelly (but not an oil-based lubricant) to avoid tearing. Oil-based lubricants may destroy the condom.
5. If, during sex, you feel that the condom has fallen off or split, then, while holding the rim of the condom at the base of the penis, withdraw from your partner.
6. After sex, withdraw quickly. As you lose your erection, the condom will loosen and seminal fluid may begin to spill.
7. Prior to discarding, check the condom for breakage.

Bottom Line: If you are going to have sex, use a latex condom with a spermicide such as nonoxynol 9. Put the condom on correctly before intercourse and dispose of it properly after intercourse. If you or your partner use no contraception, then after one year of regular intercourse, there is a 90 percent chance that your girlfriend will become pregnant.

Emergency contraception: Women who have had unprotected intercourse or have had a condom rupture during intercourse can receive emergency contraception which is also referred to as the morning after pill. These hormone pills, which are prescribed by a medical provider, must be started within 72 hours of the unprotected intercourse. They are very effective in preventing pregnancy but not sexually transmitted disease. It is thought that they act by preventing either ovulation, the release of an egg, fertilization, or implantation of the fertilized egg. Emergency contraception should not be a usual method of contraception.

SEXUALLY TRANSMITTED DISEASES

Sexually transmitted diseases (STDs) are not a new phenomenon. More than 3, 500 years ago, there were reports of STDs. Hippocrates described painful genital sores and difficulty with urination.

We know a lot more about sexually transmitted diseases now than we did 20 or even 10 years ago. Unfortunately, this greater awareness has not translated into action. On the contrary, greater numbers of male teens now have contracted one or more STDs. But it is not too late. There are

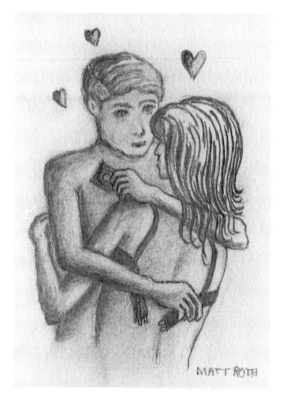

All too often, male teens do not use condoms that would help protect them from sexually transmitted diseases.

ways to reduce the probability that you will become infected. We know that there are certain factors that increase the chance that a male teen will acquire a STD.

- All too often, male teens do not use condoms that would help protect them from STDs.
- Large numbers of male teens feel invulnerable to disease and are willing to take risks.
- The use of drugs with sex or drugs for sex places males in a riskier situation for STDs.
- Many males are not monogamous. They may have multiple sex partners at one time, increasing their risk of contracting STDs.
- Male teens arc having sex at younger ages than they did years ago. That creates the potential for them to have more sexual experiences and more partners, both of which increase the risk of STDs.

For at least the past 15 years, the government has mounted an aggressive educational campaign to promote the use of barrier contraceptives such as condoms as a way to prevent Human Immunodeficiency Virus (HIV). If the campaign were successful, then we would expect a decline in the incidence of certain sexually transmitted diseases. However, it was recently reported that between the late 1970s and the early 1990s, the number of cases of genital herpes had grown significantly. For your protection, you need to use barrier methods and also know about the more common STDs.

Genital Herpes

Not that long ago, a 17-year-old male patient came to me with painful sores in his mouth. Though he was not sexually active with his partner, he did admit to performing oral sex on her. While he reported that she had no symptoms of an STD, a culture from one of the sores found that he had acquired genital herpes.

Up to 25 percent of women have genital herpes infections. Many have no idea that they are infected. About 18 percent of males have the infection.

If you acquire a genital herpes infection, you will develop painful sores on your penis, lips, mouth, or some other body parts. These are caused by a virus. *Once you are infected, you will always carry the virus*. With or without medical treatment, the sores will heal within three weeks. In all probability, the sores will reappear in the future. An examination and certain laboratory tests will enable your medical provider to diagnose a herpes infection. There are antiviral medications such as acyclovir, famciclovir, or valacyclovir which may be used to shorten an outbreak of the infection as well as prevent future outbreaks.

Now here is the key: By using a condom prior to intercourse, you may well prevent a herpes infection. Knowing your partner well and avoiding direct contact between your lips and her genitals is also important. Some males place plastic wrap or a nonlubricated condom which has been cut down the middle over the female's genitals prior to oral-genital sex.

If you do acquire herpes, it is your obligation to notify your current and any future sex partners that you are infected.

Gonorrhea

One of my 16-year-old male patients had painful urination and a yellow discharge from his penis that resembled pus. He mentioned that he had a new female sex partner, and they had had sexual intercourse about three days before he became ill. I tested the pus and determined that he had gonorrhea.

Gonorrhea is caused by bacteria. If you do not use a condom, after one act of intercourse with an infected female, you have a 30 percent chance of acquiring this disease. After 10 acts of intercourse with an infected female, you have very close to a 100 percent chance. In other words, when you're sexually exposed to an infected female, it is relatively easy to contract gonorrhea. The infection may involve your urethra, epididymis, prostate, anus, or mouth. Typically the infection starts in your urethra, which is the tube that conveys urine from your bladder through your penis to the outside. The infection can track back to the epididymis, which is a small sac overlying the top of each testicle or to your prostate, which straddles your bladder. If you have oral or anal sex, then gonorrhea can cause infection in those areas. Generally, you will have pain and discharge if you do acquire a gonococcal infection. Gonorrhea will not go away. So it is necessary to see your medical provider as soon as possible. The test for this STD is relatively easy. Treatment consists of antibiotics, which may be administered by mouth or injection.

If you are not treated, and you have sex without a condom, after one sex act, your female partner has a 70 percent change of getting gonorrhea. Females who contract gonorrhea may become seriously ill, experiencing pelvic infections, abscesses, and possible infertility.

If you are diagnosed with gonorrhea, you need to tell your partner. You can avoid infecting your partner by using a condom with nonoxynol 9 when having intercourse.

Chlamydia

Chlamydia is far more common than many people realize. During routine physicals, medical providers often find evidence of this STD in high-risk patients.

I recall a 16-year-old patient who was feeling perfectly fine and who came in for a sports physical. Still, as a precaution, I ordered some blood tests and a urine test. I was surprised to find white blood cells in his urine.

I asked him to return for a second visit, and we further discussed his sexual history and sexual partners. I then tested him for gonorrhea and chlamydia. His test for chlamydia, a bacterial infection that may cause inflammation of the epididymis, urethra, and prostate, was positive, and I treated him for that STD.

The most frequent candidates for chlamydia are males younger than 20 years old, who have begun new sexual relationships that are less than two months old, and who do not use condoms. Up to 27 percent of high risk women and 35 percent of high risk men may have chlamydia. Frequently, males have few or no symptoms. Some have a scant discharge from the urethra.

To determine if chlamydia is present, your medical provider will take a sample from the urethra. The treatment is relatively easy—an oral antibiotic.

If you have chlamydia, you need to tell your partner so she can be treated. While many women have no symptoms, untreated chlamydia in women may lead to pelvic infections and infertility. Properly using a latex condom with nonoxynol 9 will help protect you and your partner from chlamydia.

Syphilis

Syphilis, a disease caused by a spirochete, which is a microorganism, has been with us for hundreds of years. The incidence of syphilis peaked in frequency among teenage males in 1989 when there were close to 2,000 reported cases among males age 15 to 19. The incidence now is lessened, but this is a serious STD.

Syphilis usually begins with a painless sore on the penis. If the lip or finger were used in sex, they may also have a sore. The sore, which is known as a chancre, appears between one and 12 weeks after a sexual encounter with an infected partner. With or without medical treatment— usually with the antibiotic penicillin—the sore will heal, but this does not mean the disease is gone.

If you are not treated for syphilis, the disease will evolve over several months into a more serious problem, including a body rash and flu-like symptoms. If you are still not treated for syphilis, the disease will transition into a quiet phase, called latency which may continue for years. After that, a far more serious tertiary syphilis may emerge, bringing on significant bone, heart, or brain problems.

Diagnosing syphilis just takes a blood test. When early-stage syphilis is caught and treated, it has no long-term consequences. It is truly unfortunate that syphilis ever develops into the more serious stages.

Most states require people who have syphilis to reveal the names of their sex partners. A government agency will contact these partners and suggest that they seek medical care. Women with internal sores may be unaware that they have syphilis. So it is imperative that they be notified. Pregnant women with syphilis may cause damage to their unborn children, so they must receive immediate treatment.

While condoms may help prevent syphilis, if the lips, tongue, or fingers have been used during sex and have had contact with syphilitic secretions, they may spread the bacteria.

Genital Warts

Recently, a 19-year-old patient came to my office complaining of growths on his penis. For several months, he had been having sexual intercourse with the same female partner. Examination showed small, fleshy, wart-like growths on the shaft of the penis. A dermatologist confirmed my impression that they were genital warts. While the patient received liquid nitrogen, a topical treatment, I am fairly certain that at some point he will be back again. It is difficult to completely eradicate from the body the papilloma viruses that cause genital warts.

Until their sex partner is diagnosed with genital warts, most males do not realize that they are also infected. So many undiagnosed males spread the disease by unsafe sexual practices. While some males get warts on their lips or tongue, warts usually occur where there is friction. Thus, the penis is most likely to be affected.

Genital warts, which are caused by many different types of viruses, are more common in individuals who are younger, do not use condoms, and have multiple sexual partners. Treatment is usually liquid nitrogen, which is much colder than ice.

Some types of genital-warts may cause cancer of the penis, vulva (the external genitals of the female), or cervix (the outlet for the female's uterus). Your best protection is to use a latex condom with nonoxynol 9.

Hepatitis B

Caused by a virus, hepatitis B is a type of liver infection that is transmitted through sexual contact. Generally, people who develop hepatitis B experience few symptoms. These would be a loss of appetite, abdominal discomfort, nausea, fever, and a yellowing of the skin and eyes (jaundice). Though most recover fairly quickly, a small percentage will develop chronic liver disease and become carriers. A carrier is able to transmit the virus to a partner during sexual contact. When hepatitis B is in a carrier state, it is extremely difficult to treat effectively. Diagnosis is made by a blood test.

Hepatitis B is prevented by a series of three immunization shots. All adolescents should receive the series. Exceptions should be rare.

Prevention includes obtaining the hepatitis B vaccine series, and using latex condoms with nonoxynol 9.

Pubic Lice (Crabs)

When the 15-year-old arrived at my office, he was in a state of total panic. He had intense itching in his crotch, and he saw bugs crawling in his pubic area. As we spoke, he told me that he had recently been having sex with a new partner. It soon became apparent that he had eggs (nits) of pubic lice in his pubic hair.

Pubic lice are transmitted when one has close contact during vaginal or anal sex. The lice are able to jump up to one inch from one partner to another. Lice are insects that have sex with one another. The females lay eggs on the pubic hair. Within days, the eggs hatch, and the louse quickly grows into the adult stage. Lice get their nourishment by biting you and sucking your blood. The painful itch is from this biting. Thankfully, lice can be killed relatively easily with certain medicated shampoos that contain an insecticide such as permethrin.

Condoms will not prevent lice infestation. You need to know your partner well before sexual contact.

The Human Immunodeficiency Virus (HIV)

Since the late 1970s, when it was first identified, HIV has received the most attention of any STD. That is largely because of the poor prognosis faced by the vast majority of those who are infected with HIV and go on to develop full-blown AIDS. There has been a tremendous public health effort to stem the tide of the disease. In some U.S. communities, this had resulted in a leveling off of the numbers of people newly diagnosed with HIV or AIDS.

When one first acquires the virus, there may be no symptoms. Eventually, as the immune system is compromised, the patient will begin to show signs of illness. But being infected with HIV is not the same as having AIDS. There are strict definitions as to what constitutes AIDS. Many more adolescents are infected with the virus than have the end result, which is termed AIDS.

As of June 1997, 1,852 U.S. male adolescents had been diagnosed with AIDS. A much higher number are infected with the virus. Of these 1,852 teens, 38 percent were hemophiliacs, 34 percent acquired AIDS through homosexual contact, 6 percent used intravenous drugs, 4 percent had blood transfusions, and 3 percent had sex with a female. The source of the virus in the remainder was not identified.

In my adolescent medicine practice, I see many male teens who are worried that they may have acquired HIV. Not too long ago, a 19-year-old male came to see me after having unprotected sex with a new female partner. Both he and his partner had been drinking excessively and were drunk. He remembered little about the encounter and did not even recall her name. He never expected to see her again and asked to be tested for HIV.

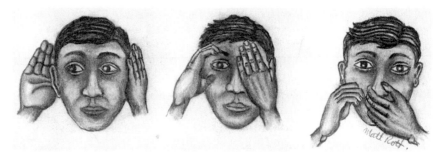

Health professionals testing for HIV guard patients' confidentiality.

There are actually two HIV blood tests that screen for antibodies to the virus. When someone is tested, the Elisa is first performed. If that test is positive, a second test, Western Blot, is automatically performed. If you have a positive result to the Elisa and the Western Blot, you have tested positive for HIV.

You should know that after you're first exposed to the virus, antibodies to HIV ordinarily take three to six months to appear. Thus, if you are exposed to HIV in January, you might not know if you were infected or not until June. If you decide to be tested, you should go to a center which has pre- and post-test counseling services. I never recommend home testing kits. Although there may be a long wait, every state has anonymous testing centers. At these centers, patients are usually given a number. When you return for the results, you give the staff your number. The results are never connected with your name and are therefore anonymous.

A positive HIV test means that you have the virus and are able to infect others through unsafe sexual practices or the sharing of intravenous drug paraphernalia.

Large numbers of health professionals are able to test teens for HIV, and the results are protected through medical confidentiality. Many states require your written approval before the results may be released to anyone.

There is absolutely no way to determine if you should be tested for HIV after risky sex. For some unfortunate teens, one risky sexual episode may lead to HIV. Others have hundreds of risky encounters and never acquire HIV. There is no way to predict your odds.

As a result, it is essential that you adopt safer sex methods with any partner. This includes knowing your partner, using barrier methods such as condoms and rubber dams, not exchanging bodily fluids such as semen or vaginal fluid, and also using a contraceptive substance, such as nonoxynol 9, which helps kill HIV.

Using substances such as alcohol and cocaine around the time of sex may lead to more risky behavior. And if you already have an STD, such as genital herpes, and engage in risky sex, then you have a still-higher chance of acquiring HIV. Because the skin barrier has been broken by the herpes infection, there are more pathways for HIV to enter the body.

The treatment of HIV is beyond the scope of this book. Nevertheless, it should be noted that there are now triple drug therapies (known as "cocktails"), which are effective in prolonging the life of patients with this disease. People use the term, "living with AIDS." But these cocktails do not work for everyone, and they sometimes have negative side effects. They are also quite expensive. A preventive vaccine is nowhere near development for public use. So HIV is one STD that must be prevented through safer sex practices.

ISSUES OF IMPORTANCE TO GAY ADOLESCENTS

It is estimated that 10 percent of adolescents struggle with issues related to sexual orientation, defined as a person's pattern of physical and emotional arousal toward other individuals. The famous researcher Alfred Kinsey felt that most people were not entirely homosexual or entirely heterosexual. Kinsey believed that the majority of people had both heterosexual and homosexual feelings. Gay teens often recall that even when they were quite young, they felt different from most of their peers. There is no scientific proof that sexual abuse, traumatic life events, or bad parenting will make a male teen gay.

Many male adolescents who experience homosexual feelings struggle with their identity. Some of these teens attempt to "correct" their feelings by avoiding stereotypical homosexual activities or escaping through substance abuse. Around ages 17–21, many gay males begin to assume their sexual identity. The last stage of homosexual identity formation is when the gay adolescent accepts his homosexuality. At this stage, same-sex love relationships and disclosure of sexual orientation to family and friends may occur.

A 17-year-old male came to my office asking for an HIV test. He stated that he had been attracted to men for years, and, in recent weeks, had several sexual relationships with older men whom he met through the Internet. When he confided this behavior to his parents, they asked him to seek medical assistance as soon as possible.

Gay male adolescents face a number of unique issues. Homophobia is prevalent almost everywhere. All too often, male teens who "appear gay" in high school endure ridicule, social isolation, and alienation. Dances and other social events may be awkward, and gay males are often threatened with violence, verbal harassment, and social stigma.

Large numbers of gay teens are depressed; some consider suicide. Tragically, too many succeed in killing themselves.

When gays confide their sexual orientation to their parents, they are sometimes greeted with rejection and abandonment. This leads to further isolation, possible hopelessness, and prostitution (further increasing the risk of contracting HIV). It is not uncommon for gay teens to turn to alcohol and drugs to relieve the stress of loneliness and family condemnation.

While some parents may disapprove of their child's gay sexual orientation at first, often blaming their own parenting skills, in time many accept their teen's gay orientation. Parents are best told about your gay sexual orientation when you have a positive feeling about it and when your relationship with them is going well.

Gay adolescent males are at risk for STDs as are straight males. This is not because they are gay. Rather, it is a result of their sexual practices. For example, unprotected anal intercourse often leads to STDs.

As a gay teen, it is very important for you to establish a good relationship with a primary care physician. I appreciate it when my patients tell me directly that they are gay. If you engage in high-risk homosexual behaviors, you must be checked periodically for STDs, immunized against hepatitis A and B, and offered emotional support. You probably already know that not all physicians are sensitive to the issues of gay male teens. If you believe that your physician is not, try to obtain the names of other physicians who are sympathetic. These names may be obtained from gay organizations, other gay teens, or knowledgeable professionals.

SEXUAL ABUSE

Sexual abuse refers to unwanted sexual activity. Abuse occurs when sexual activity is forced on another person either against that person's will or—if that person is young or impaired—incapable of giving consent.

Surveys show that one out of every six males is sexually abused before the age of 19. That statistic may be far too low. Partly because of the stigma society places on homosexual abuse, many cases of abuse in males are not reported. You should be assured that there is no relationship between homosexual abuse and homosexual orientation. In other words, if you are not already gay, you will not become gay as a result of homosexual abuse.

Abused males are victimized in several ways. First, for a male to acknowledge that he is a victim implies that he is not manly. In addition, our culture encourages males not to admit pain. Instead, they should deny it. Sexually victimized males believe that since our society contends that males should fight back, they may be blamed for the abuse. Males may not recognize the abuse or be too intimidated by an authoritarian or powerful abuser. Then the abuse will go unreported.

Male adolescents and young adults who never reported their sexual abuse may carry a tremendous psychological burden. If you have been a victim of sexual abuse, you should discuss this with your physician, a school counselor, or a social worker. Individual and group counseling as well as self-help groups are available to assist you. If the perpetrator is a family member, then that person must be identified and treated before the family can be reunited. Male sexual abuse crosses all social bounds. It is not limited to any race, religion, age, nationality, socioeconomic class, or sexual orientation. But it is important for you to come forward as soon as possible and disclose what is happening.

ACQUAINTANCE RAPE

Forcing someone you know to have sexual intercourse against her or his will is acquaintance rape, also known as date rape. It is a form of sexual assault. Generally, males are not the victims; they are usually the perpetrators. Women are the most frequent victims.

Because of gender stereotypes, males may erroneously assume that women want intercourse. The following actions should *not* be interpreted as signals that a woman wants to have sex:

- Drinking
- Kissing
- Wearing sexually provocative clothing
- Agreeing to come to your room
- Previous acts of intercourse

As a male adolescent, it is imperative that you understand that if a woman says, "No," to your sexual advantages, you must not attempt to have sex with her. Never force sex on an unwilling partner. Never use substances such as rohypnol, alcohol, or GBH (liquid ecstasy) on a partner to induce her to have sex. (See chapter 6 for more information.) Learn to control your sexual impulses.

You should realize that victims of acquaintance rape may press charges. Most males involved in sexual assault have been drinking, so you should not drink to the extent that it dulls your senses. In fact, excess alcohol may dull your sexual feeling and cause the loss of an erection. Obviously, the best and most satisfactory sex is consensual between partners. You should strive for an appropriate sexual relationship.

ADDITIONAL INFORMATION

Centers for Disease Control
National STD Hotline
800–227–8922

Centers for Disease Control
National AIDS Hotline
800–342-AIDS
800–344-SIDA (Spanish)

Herpes Resource Center
800–230–6039

REFERENCES

Centers for Disease Control and Prevention. "1998 Guidelines for Treatment of Sexually Transmitted Disease." Atlanta, Ga.: Government Printing Office, 1997.
Centers for Disease Control and Prevention. "Youth Risk Behavior Surveillance—United States, 1997." Atlanta, Ga.: Government Printing Office, 1998.
Centers for Disease Control and Prevention. "Youth Risk Behavior Surveillance—National Alternative High School Youth Risk Behavior Survey, United States, 1998." Atlanta, Ga.: Government Printing Office, 1999.
Winikoff, Beverly, and Suzanne Wymelenberg. *The Whole Truth about Contraception.* Washington, D.C.: The Joseph Henry Press, 1997.

6

Alcohol, Tobacco, and Drugs

In late September 1997, Scott Krueger, a brilliant, handsome, 18-year-old freshman from Orchard Park, New York, was found unconscious in his room at a Massachusetts Institute of Technology fraternity. Although he was rushed to a Boston hospital, doctors were unable to save him. After three days in a coma, his life support was disconnected. Within minutes, he died.

Scott's coma was not the result of some fluke of nature or medical tragedy. Rather, it was caused directly by alcohol. Scott had been drinking excessively. In all probability, he vomited and then inhaled his own vomitus, causing him to suffocate. The suffocation resulted in severe brain damage. Scott's family will forever live with the knowledge that his death was completely and entirely preventable. It was the senseless waste of a life that had so much promise.

Unfortunately, Scott is not alone. Every year, adolescents die from the abuse of alcohol and other drugs. Yet, it is a reality many parents find hard to acknowledge. But denying the truth will not make it go away. By the time the vast majority of males complete their adolescence, they will have used some type of harmful drug.

Of course, there are a wide variety of drugs. Some may cause immediate damage or even death. Others take their toll over time. Some are illegal for people of certain ages. Others are legal or illegal for everyone. This chapter will describe drugs that fall into all these categories—alcohol, tobacco, marijuana, cocaine, heroin, anabolic steroids, amphetamines, LSD, designer drugs, PCP, and inhalants.

Why are male adolescents drawn to drugs? The following are at least some of the reasons:

- Adolescence is a time of exploration and experimentation.
- Male adolescents often feel they are invincible.
- Adolescent males are particularly susceptible to peer pressure and do not know how to say "no" and still remain on good terms with their friends.
- Parents are permissive about drug use.
- Parents use drugs, and adolescents are modeling their behavior.
- Adolescents may be influenced by role models, such as sport stars, who use drugs.
- Adolescents may be directly and indirectly influenced by the mass media.

Let's examine this last point. A beer ad in a popular magazine shows a group of attractive young men and women drinking beer while playing volleyball on the beach. The ad skillfully implies that everyone drinks beer. Moreover, the subliminal message conveyed by the ad is this: Since one may successfully play a sport while drinking beer, beer drinking must be safe. As an added plus, drinking beer will just about guarantee acceptance by your peers.

Since beer manufacturers are out to sell their products, their advertising fails to note a few key points. Drinking beer will impair your ability to play sports. When you drink beer and play sports, you may hurt yourself or someone else. The ad does not suggest that it is perfectly okay to party in a crowd without drinking beer. In fact, it is not necessary to drink simply because others are drinking.

Statistics from the U.S. government Youth Risk Behavior Surveillance survey compiled in 1995 are truly startling:

- 72 percent of high school males have used tobacco and 35 percent currently use it.
- 81 percent of high school males have used alcohol and 53 percent currently use it.
- 45 percent of high school males have used marijuana and 28 percent currently use it.
- 9 percent of high school males have used cocaine and 4 percent currently use it.
- 5 percent of high school males have used illegal steroids.

While it is illegal for adolescents to use the vast majority of drugs covered in this chapter, I will refrain from a discussion of the legal implications. As a physician, it is my role to teach, not to pass judgment. Still, I hope that once you have learned more about drugs and their potential negative health consequences, you will decide to exercise caution.

ALCOHOL

We've all seen the images on television. Rowdy male teens drinking large pitchers of beer at a high school or college party. Clearly, they have one goal—to get drunk as quickly as possible. Supposedly, such behavior is fun and fosters camaraderie among friends. That is why teens who choose to drink are drawn to other teens who choose to drink. But teens who do not want to drink may also be influenced by peer pressure and drink just to "fit in."

Several other factors play a role in teenage drinking as well. Do the parents of teenage drinkers abuse alcohol? Parents who abuse alcohol often have children who abuse alcohol. Is alcohol readily available in the home? If there is a plentiful supply of alcohol, it may be easy to sneak a bottle or two without anyone knowing. Do the teens have access to adults who are willing to buy alcohol for them? Most teens are able to find someone who would gladly purchase alcohol and make a few dollars in the process. And how influenced are the teens by the mass media, which glorifies and romanticizes alcohol? Don't ever underestimate the power of advertising.

So what is wrong with alcohol and why is there reason for concern about teens who drink? To understand the consequences of drinking, let's first look at what alcohol does when it enters your body. When you drink alcohol, it rapidly passes from your mouth to your stomach and small intestine. If you have not eaten any solid food, it travels even faster. Within moments, it enters your bloodstream. Passing throughout the body, it is metabolized by the liver. Heavy drinkers are able to tolerate more alcohol than light drinkers and are therefore able to drink more before becoming drunk. Alcohol also increases urination, which may lead to dehydration and some hangover symptoms.

Alcohol depresses the central nervous system. Thus, drinkers initially feel more relaxed, often becoming more sociable and talkative. As the drinking continues, however, that changes. At higher blood-alcohol levels, your speech may become slurred and your coordination diminishes. At even higher levels, you may vomit, lose consciousness, or black out. Every year, teens die as a direct result of drinking. They may drive under the influence. Alcohol-related car crashes are the leading cause of death among teens. Or they may fall or experience cardiac or respiratory arrest from excessive blood-alcohol levels.

In European countries, where alcohol often accompanies meals, teens generally learn to drink responsibly. Because parents teach their teens to respect alcohol, the problems commonly seen in the United States are far less prevalent in Europe. In addition, Europeans view drunkenness with disdain. It is not socially acceptable.

One of my patients, whom I had known for 18 years, had never had a drink before entering college. While attending one of his first parties, he drank excessively with his friends. That is all he remembered about the night. His friends told him that he began to vomit and blacked out. They transported him to the emergency department of a major Boston hospital. After awakening the next day, he vowed that he would never again drink recklessly. Thus far he has honored that personal pledge.

It is important to understand that if you choose to use alcohol irresponsibly, you may endanger yourself and others. Thus, if you become drunk and have forcible sex with a date, you will be held accountable. After all, you remember almost nothing. It all seemed like such a blur. But that is not how the criminal justice system views what you did. Just because you were drunk and did not know what you were doing, you may still be charged with a criminal offense, such as date rape.

To discourage driving after drinking, most states have enacted laws placing strict limits on drinking and driving. If there is a trace of alcohol on a teen's breath, he will lose his license. For example, a blood-alcohol level of .02 percent, which a 170 pound male may have after only one beer, is considered legally drunk for teens in some states. If you live in one of those states with a zero tolerance policy toward drunk driving, and you are stopped and found to be legally drunk, you will immediately lose your driver's license.

If someone you know has been drinking and has one or more of the following symptoms, then there may be a medical emergency. You should seek help or call 911 immediately:

- cold, clammy, pale, or bluish skin
- breathing fewer than eight times per minute
- passed out or cannot be awakened
- vomiting while sleeping
- no pulse or breathing

TOBACCO

I currently care for a 17-year-old junior in high school who smokes two packs of cigarettes a day. His teeth are yellow; he has lost his edge in sports, and he smells of tobacco. He maintains that he is unable to stop smoking. But he is hoping to reduce the number of cigarettes he smokes. Though he admits to an addiction, he refuses counseling and says that he cannot afford to purchase medications that will help curb his habit. He regrets that he began smoking and that he is physically and psychologically unable to stop. Conceivably, he could continue smoking for decades, until smoking totally ravages his body and he dies an untimely death.

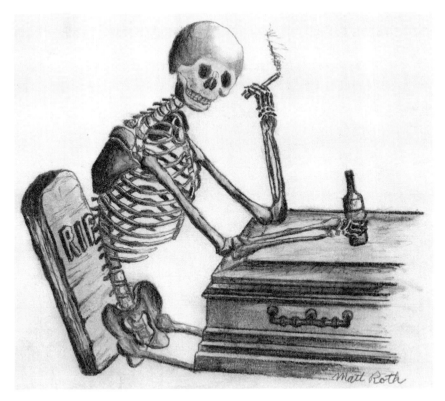

Irresponsible heavy drinking, as well as tobacco use, can ravage the body and can lead to an untimely death.

All forms of tobacco—cigarettes, cigars, pipe tobacco, and chewing tobacco—contain nicotine, a central nervous system stimulant. Over a period of time, the regular use of nicotine will lead to true drug dependence. In fact, long-term users of tobacco may experience profound withdrawal when they attempt to stop.

Several generations ago, people were generally unaware of the negative effects of tobacco. Today, that is no longer true. There is absolutely no reason for teens to begin using any tobacco products.

We all know that there is a relationship between lung cancer and inhaled cigarette smoke. Even the cigarette companies have admitted that. But, as a teen, you may not be concerned about developing cancer in your 50s, 60s, or 70s. From your perspective, that seems too far into the future for any serious concern. On the other hand, you may wish to know that tobacco products have more immediate consequences. Chewing tobacco causes mouth lesions, even in younger people. It is not uncommon for a person in his 20s who chews tobacco to develop mouth cancer. If you smoke tobacco, you may become short of breath. If you strive to be an athlete, the use of tobacco products may reduce your level of performance. You may develop a smoker's cough and be more susceptible to respiratory illness. And if you are an asthmatic and you smoke, your condition will worsen.

Then there are the social negatives to smoking. People who use tobacco have a distinctive odor to their breath, hair, and clothes. Frequently, their teeth are stained yellow. If they smoke inside, their furnishings will smell of tobacco. And tobacco is expensive. A pack of cigarettes costs more than $2.75 and a tin of chewing tobacco is about $5.00.

Finally, increasingly, society is making life difficult for smokers. Many workplaces will not allow smoking inside the building. Large numbers of restaurants are smoke-free, as are airline flights within the United States. People who are found to be smoking in an airline bathroom will be severely fined. It is no longer cool to smoke. Beside the cost, inconvenience, and social non-acceptability of tobacco products, if you choose to use them, you will hurt your body physically and mentally. There is no reason to use tobacco products.

MARIJUANA

Recently, one of my high school patients was preparing for a trip with his school orchestra. Excitedly, he told me that they were scheduled to give several concerts to young audiences in Europe. It would, he believed, be the highlight of his high school career.

Regrettably, before the trip, he was driving around in a car with several friends. The friends, but not my patient, were smoking marijuana (pot). When they were stopped by the police, my patient denied that he had smoked pot. However, when a urine test was done, marijuana metabolites were found. My patient did not realize that secondhand smoke may also result in a positive urine test. So even though he was not smoking pot, he inhaled the secondhand smoke from his friends. He should have been keeping different company. He was suspended from school, and he was not allowed to go on the trip. Whenever I see him, he continues to express regret over the incident.

Marijuana, which contains a psychoactive chemical called THC, is a mixture of the green, brown or gray dried, shredded flowers and leaves of the Cannabis sativa plant. There are several ways to use marijuana. It may be rolled into a cigarette, called a joint, and smoked. It may also be brewed in a tea. In some instances it is eaten. When smoked, users inhale the smoke deeply and hold it as long as possible in their lungs. The chemical THC is readily absorbed into the bloodstream, and it quickly travels to the brain. Though most users report that they experience a sense of euphoria, some report episodes of panic, flashbacks, depersonalization (where one loses his self-identity), and hallucinations, especially among individuals who have previously used LSD.

Since marijuana may alter judgment and delay reaction time, it could affect your ability to drive. Your capacity to study could be hampered because it reduces short-term memory. And the chemicals in the smoke may compromise athletic performance. If you are in a situation where you may be tested for marijuana—such as in an athletic competition—you should be aware that traces of marijuana stay in your body for up to a month. Furthermore, as in the case of my patient, if you have inhaled secondhand marijuana smoke, your urine may test positive for marijuana. So it is best not to be near anyone who is smoking marijuana. Chronic abuse of marijuana may lead to the diminution of male sex hormones, which may result in lower sperm production and impotence or an inability to perform sexually. That is quite a sobering thought for a healthy, young male.

COCAINE

Cocaine, an extremely addictive and powerful brain stimulant, is extracted from the leaves of the coca plant. Always illegal, it is sold on the street in two forms. The first type is a white crystalline substance, cocaine hydrochloride, which can be snorted in your nose or dissolved in water and injected into a vein. The second variety, crack cocaine, has been chemically processed and may be smoked as chips, chunks, or rocks.

Cocaine users report experiencing a surge of energy, confidence, and intense pleasure. When cocaine is shot into the vein, they get an instantaneous high. The high from smoking cocaine comes more slowly. But the high lasts only briefly and generally diminishes in about 20 minutes. As cocaine leaves the brain, there is a crash, characterized by depression, irritability, and fatigue.

I recall one of my patients who was an excellent student during the first two years of high school. Then, as a junior, his grades began to decline. Soon, he was failing courses. He became antisocial and lost many of his friends. He was also chronically short of money. Eventually, his parents insisted that he be examined. Though he initially protested, he finally agreed. During his physical examination, I noticed some erosion of the skin on his nasal septum (the wall that divides the nasal passages into two sections). When I told him what I had found, he admitted that he was using cocaine. I referred him to a substance abuse specialist. His recovery was long and slow and had many stops, starts, and curves.

It is an understatement to say that those who use cocaine place themselves at serious risk. The mood swings and depression brought on by cocaine use may lead to problems coping with everyday life, work, school, athletics, and sex. Obtaining the money to pay for this addictive drug may

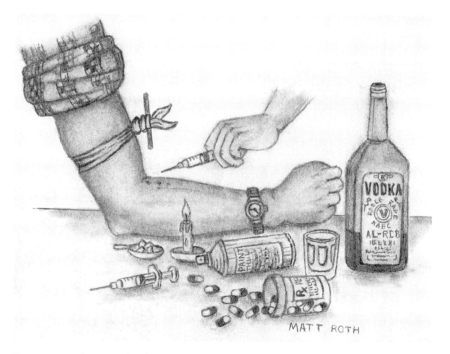

Some teens abuse multiple substances that can be a great risk to their health.

force users into risky sexual behavior. Males have been known to become prostitutes for other males in order to obtain money to purchase more cocaine. Those who shoot cocaine into their veins are at risk for acquiring HIV or hepatitis from dirty "works" (syringes and needles). Cocaine has destroyed many lives. It is imperative that you stay far away from it.

ANABOLIC STEROIDS

Not that long ago, a very bright 20-year-old man came to me with disturbing symptoms. His testicles were shrinking. Moreover, he was increasingly losing interest in sex. I was not shocked. I had heard this complaint before. Shrinking testicles is common in men 65 years of age and older and in younger men who use anabolic steroids. My patient admitted to using anabolic steroids. He was hoping to build muscle mass. Instead, he had shrinking testicles and a lessened desire for sex. Immediately, he discontinued his steroid use. We are still waiting to see how long it will take for his testicles and feelings about sex to return to normal.

Anabolic steroids are synthetic hormones closely related to the male sex hormone testosterone. Although there are legitimate medical reasons

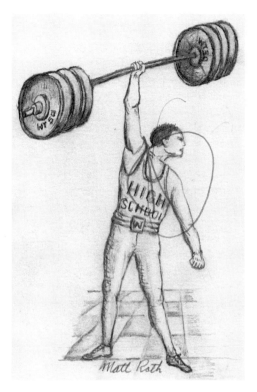

Although there are legitimate medical reasons for the use of anabolic steroids, all too often they are used illegally by athletes and body builders who feel that steroids will give them a competitive advantage or improve the way they look. Using steroids may have serious negative side effects.

for the use of anabolic steroids, all too often they are illegally used by athletes and body builders who feel that steroids will give them a competitive advantage or improve the way they look.

What is not well known is that anabolic steroids may have serious negative side effects. If you take anabolic steroids while you are still growing, they may cause the growth centers in your bones to shut down, thereby stunting your growth. You will not grow to your full potential. Abuse of anabolic steroids may cause your testicles to shrink and that could affect sexual performance. Your skin may break out in a severe case of acne, and you might become prematurely bald. All in all, unless a physician has prescribed anabolic steroids for a specific medical problem, stay far away from them.

AMPHETAMINES

Amphetamines go by various names. They are called speed, meth, crank, crystal, ice, uppers, black beauties, pep pills, copilots, bumblebees, hearts, benzedrine, dexedrine, and footballs. While the names may differ, amphetamines, which may be taken by mouth, smoked, injected, or snorted, all stimulate the central nervous system, producing a sense of well-being and energy. Users note a release of social inhibitions and say they feel clever, competent, and powerful. Though such feelings might sound appealing, there is another side to amphetamines.

Amphetamines may cause transient high blood pressure, fever, racing heart beats, rapid breathing, dilated pupils, seizures, and heart-rhythm disturbances. Chronic use of amphetamines may produce a type of mental disturbance similar to schizophrenia. Teens may become paranoid, have hallucinations, and develop violent and erratic behavior.

Crystalline methamphetamine is a twist on amphetamines. Known on the street as ice, speed, or crystal, it is a highly purified crystalline form of amphetamine, which is smoked, snorted, swallowed, or injected. The side effects are similar to those seen with amphetamines. These are dangerous drugs, unless prescribed by a physician for a medical problem.

LSD

Several years ago, on a hot and humid day in July, I received a call notifying me that a student had fallen out of a building. Having fallen several stories, his vital organs were crushed, and he was dead on impact. In time, it became apparent that he had taken LSD, also known as acid, and was on a bad "trip" when the fall occurred. It is well known that LSD trips may be exceedingly violent. LSD (which stands for lysergic acid diethylamide) may completely distort a person's perception and sense of time. It may cause people to believe they have unusual powers, such as the ability to fly. Some people become paranoid and think they are being pursued. And LSD causes the senses to become more pronounced. For example, smells may be stronger, visual images more vivid, and the sense of touch more acute.

LSD is available in several forms, including tablets (microdots) and gelatin squares (windowpanes). In addition, paper may be soaked with LSD to form "blotters," which are chewed.

Although LSD is not addictive, users may have a "bad trip" in which they experience panic, disorientation, loss of control, confusion, suspicion, and anxiety. Even those who no longer use LSD may have flashbacks. Like the student who had fallen out of the building, the literature contains reports of numerous people who have died or committed suicide during trips or flashbacks. There are good reasons for this drug to be illegal.

HEROIN

Having graduated from college, one of my former patients remained in the Boston area where he lived and worked. One day, I was stunned to receive a report that he was found dead in his apartment. Apparently, he had accidentally overdosed on heroin. His ongoing addiction to that drug had inadvertently resulted in his premature death.

Heroin, a powder that varies in color from white to dark brown, is a highly addictive drug that is most often shot into a vein (mainlined). When injected, it reaches the brain in 15 to 30 seconds. Heroin—also known as smack, horse, junk, and dope—may be smoked or inhaled through the nose. Reportedly, it generates an intensely pleasureful high. But to maintain this high, users require increasing amounts of this illegal drug.

The many dangers of heroin include physical addiction, sudden death from respiratory arrest, and heart disturbances. Those who inject heroin run the risk of contracting HIV and hepatitis from dirty needles and syringes. Severe infections, including those affecting the heart values, are not uncommon. And the heroin habit is expensive. Too often, teens prostitute themselves or become involved in other illegal activities to support their addiction. Withdrawal from heroin is excruciatingly painful. Professional help is required. Clearly, any experimentation with this drug is dangerous and potentially deadly.

DESIGNER DRUGS

Designer drugs are synthetic modifications of commonly abused drugs. Illicit laboratories synthesize them for recreational use. Because they are created by underground "chemists," they may not necessarily be listed by the federal government as illegal. Some designer drugs are related to opiates, such as heroin, and amphetamines. But as drugs synthesized in clandestine laboratories, they may be extremely dangerous.

Ecstasy, also known as MDMA or Adam, is an example of a designer drug that acts as a stimulant and a hallucinogen. Users take Ecstasy to stimulate their central nervous system. But Ecstasy also distorts the user's sense of well-being. It reduces the level of serotonin, an important brain chemical, for up to two weeks. Ecstasy users often have the desire to touch others and move around; some participate in all-night dance parties known as "raves." Yet Ecstasy brings on severe toxic reactions, such as elevated body temperature and dehydration, and has caused numerous deaths.

PCP

During my training in adolescent medicine, I had a 16-year-old patient who overdosed on PCP (phencyclidine). Sadly, he went into a psychotic state, and he was committed to a mental hospital for long-term treatment. In time, he was released. But his personality was forever changed.

Surprisingly, the origins of PCP—also known as angel dust, rocket fuel, or dust—are rather harmless. Initially, PCP was designed as an animal anesthetic. Then in 1963, physicians began using it as a human anesthetic. When it was found to cause agitation, hallucinations, and seizures, its use was discontinued.

PCP is a white powder that has a bitter taste. It may be snorted, smoked, or eaten. Users report mixed reactions. It causes them to feel stimulated or depressed, and it may trigger hallucinations. Other side effects include paranoia, psychosis, aggressive behavior, detachment, depression, seizures, coma, and death. Medical treatment may involve the use of restraints, placement in a dark room, and, sometimes, prolonged hospitalization. Since PCP may be added to marijuana, LSD, and methamphetamine, people may unknowingly use it. That makes it even more worrisome.

INHALANTS

As ordinary household items, inhalants are not illegal. But they were manufactured to serve some household function, not to be inhaled.

To get high, the user inhales or sniffs these products. If the substance is solid, it is placed in a paper or plastic bag and then inhaled. Liquids are usually inhaled directly from the container. The inhalants slow down certain body functions so the users may feel stimulated, disoriented, giddy, lightheaded, or even out of control. Frequently, users will feel nauseous and vomit. Users have been known to pass out and become oxygen deprived. In some cases, severe brain damage and impaired physical and mental functioning have resulted.

I vividly recall the case of a student who was inhaling nitrous oxide using a plastic tent. The individual who was supposed to watch him left the room for a few minutes. Upon returning, the non-user found his friend dead from suffocation and lack of oxygen.

Rohypnol, also known as roofies or the date rape drug, has been popular among teens. It has been erroneously viewed as a "safe" drug of abuse and that it cannot be detected by urine drug testing. Taken orally, often with alcohol or other drugs, rohypnol causes memory impairment, drowsiness, confusion, dizziness, and visual disturbances. Males who secretly administer it to women in their drinks have taken advantage of its effects to sexually assault woman. The women quickly develop fatigue and memory impairment and cannot stop or recall a sexual assault.

POLYSUBSTANCE ABUSE

About three years ago, while he was still in high school, one of my patients began using marijuana and cocaine. It did not take long for him to begin drinking alcohol. Soon, his grades fell, and he had promiscuous sexual relations with females he could not remember the day after. Finally, he started to smoke tobacco. At first, he smoked only a few cigarettes a day. After several months, he was a chain smoker.

Eventually, he was admitted to a hospital's detox unit. It has taken him two years to rebuild his life—and he is only 19. Having dropped out of college after only one term, he has a decent-paying but menial job. He regularly attends Alcoholic Anonymous meetings and has a new girlfriend who is sober. Thanks to medications and therapy, he no longer uses drugs.

He has been most challenged in his effort to stop smoking cigarettes. For several months he chewed nicotine gum. But he said it tasted terrible. He hasn't been able to stop craving cigarettes, especially in certain social situations or when waiting for the train to commute to his job. He finds himself drawn to the attractive cigarette advertising in magazines.

Still, he is finally starting to feel better about himself. Through family, friends, medical care, AA, and sheer faith, he has halted his polysubstance abuse, and he profoundly regrets the day he began.

From the material presented in this chapter you may readily understand that drugs have significant negative consequences for you and your acquaintances. I hope you will decide that the potential serious side effects are not worth the momentary high. If you do, you may save yourself a lifetime of unnecessary problems or even premature death.

> Six-forty in the evening on September 29, 1997, a life is over. Having completed for the second time in the day a battery of tests to determine if any brain function persisted and finding only silence, I disconnected Scott Krueger from his ventilator and left him with his family to say their final good-bye.
>
> As I walked into Scott's room for the last time, I focused on his younger brother who sat at the bedside. The pain on his face was almost more than I could bear. I could imagine the love and admiration he held for Scott, the good times they had shared in the past but which were now stolen from him. He is only 14 and the shock of this tragedy will likely stay with him for the rest of his life. He will have to grow up a little sooner, and he will have to grow up more alone than he should be.
>
> —Richard M. Schwartzstein, M.D.
> "The Wellesley Townsman," October 23, 1997

FURTHER INFORMATION

National Clearinghouse for Alcohol and Drug Information
1–800–729–6686
http://www.health.org/

National Institute on Drug Abuse
http://www.nida.nih.gov/

National Center on Addiction and Substance Abuse
http://www.casacolumbia.org/

Alcoholics Anonymous
http://www.alcoholics-anonymous.org/

Narcotics Anonymous
http://users.aol.com/na4napa/na1.html

Marijuana Anonymous
http://www.marijuana-anonymous.org/

Resource to Quit Smoking
http://www.quitnet.org/

American Council for Drug Education
1–800–488–DRUG

National Council for Alcoholism and Drug Dependence
1–800–622–2255

REFERENCES

Centers for Disease Control and Prevention. "Youth Risk Behavior Surveillance, National College Health Risk Behavior Survey—United States, 1995." Atlanta, Ga.: Government Printing Office, 1997.

Centers for Disease Control and Prevention. "Youth Risk Behavior Surveillance—United States, 1997." Atlanta, Ga.: Government Printing Office, 1998.

Drug Enforcement Administration Website *http://usdoj.gov/dea* January 22, 2000.

Hingson, R., T. Heeren, and M. Winter. *Lower Legal Blood Alcohol Limits for Young Drivers*. Public Health Reports, 1994. 109: 738–744.

Massachusetts Institute of Technology, Medical Department. "Alcohol—Just the Facts." Cambridge, Mass., 1998.

National Institute on Alcohol Abuse and Alcoholism. "Youth Drinking: Risk Factors and Consequences." Alcohol Alert, July 1997.

7

Sports Injuries and Sports Medicine

Teens with any body type can participate in sports. There are three body types called endomorph, ectomorph, and mesomorph as well as individuals who are tall and short in stature. Endomorph refers to a body that which has a soft roundness, an accumulation of fat, and large trunk and thighs. A mesomorph, in contrast, has a preponderance of muscle with a hard rectangular physique. An individual with an ectomorphic body type has a more linear appearance with thin muscles and less fat. Teens with any body type can succeed in sports, but all body types are susceptible to injuries.

SPORTS INJURIES

If you participate in sports, there is a fairly good chance that at some point you will experience a sports-related injury. While it is important to take as many precautions as possible and to wear protective equipment, you may still be hurt. Consider the following scenarios:

- You are running with the football toward your high school's goal post when you are suddenly clipped from behind by a member of the opposing team. As you fall, you twist your right knee. You feel a pop followed by excruciating pain. Still, you clutch the ball and fall over the goal line. As you limp to the locker room, your knee begins to swell. Later, you learn that you have a torn meniscus, which is a cushion of tissue between the bones of the knee joint, and that you are out for the season.

- It is the biggest cross-country race of the season. You have been training for months. But after the first mile, you have trouble breathing. Your pace slows,

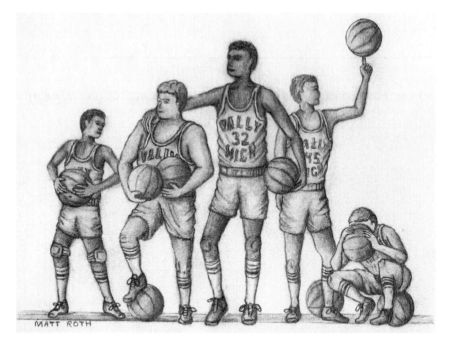

Teens with any body type can participate in sports.

and your breathing becomes labored. Unfortunately, you are forced to stop. Your doctor diagnoses exercise-induced asthma.

- You notice a painful rash with little blisters on your chest in the area where you were bruised during a match. It looks quite different from the acne on your face. In fact, it closely resembles the rash your wrestling opponent had on his chest last week. You have acquired herpes gladiatorum.

Almost any part of your body may be hurt in a sports injury. We will examine these injuries based on their location in the body.

Skin

Stretch Marks

One of my patients, a 16-year-old male rower, came to see me because he was concerned about the red marks on his back. He was in good health and the marks were not painful. Upon examination, I determined that he had stretch marks caused by the increase in muscle mass from exercise and the constant pulling on his skin from rowing. While they may be unsightly, stretch marks are harmless.

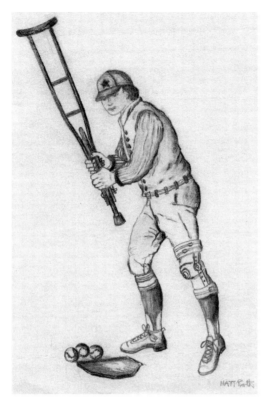

If you participate in sports, there is a fairly good chance that at some point you will experience a sports-related injury. It is important to take as many precautions as possible and to wear protective equipment.

Calluses and Corns

Calluses, or areas of thickened skin, are generally caused by inappropriate friction or pressure. While they are frequently seen on the feet, gymnasts and golfers often have them on their hands. They may be prevented by protecting the skin from friction and pressure.

Corns are calluses that are painful. Almost always found on the feet, they are a response to friction and pressure. They can and should be removed.

Blisters

Typically caused by fiction and pressure, blisters are a collection of fluid under the skin. Most often, they are found on the feet. If you tend to get blisters in a certain area, you should keep that area moist with a lubricant such as petroleum jelly. Also, if blisters appear on your feet, be sure to wear well-fitted shoes.

Bleeding

During sports, bleeding into the skin may occur under a variety of circumstances. For example, direct contact or collision with another player may cause bleeding. Bursting of blood vessels may occur after overuse of muscles or from a twisting injury. When a player steps on a toenail, there could be bleeding under the nail. Since there is very little space under the nail, that type of bleeding may be quite painful. The pressure and pain may be relieved by drilling a hole into the nail.

Bloody blisters and bruises (or contusions) are commonly seen in collision sports such as football as well as contact sports such as basketball. Recovery is often accelerated by supportive therapy, such as RICE (rest, ice, compression, elevation). Tennis and basketball players are prone to bruising and bleeding under the nails of the great and second toes. Black heel, or bleeding into the heel, is seen in athletes who play sports where there are sudden stops. Thick socks and a small bandage may be protective.

Abrasions

In males, abrasions, or the wearing away of skin due to injury, are probably the most frequent sports injury. Chafing is the skin's response to mechanical irritation. Abrasions may be caused by wrestling mats, artificial turf burn, dirt, cinders, or a variety of other agents. For example, an inappropriately fitting protective cup may cause chafing in the groin. Prevention includes the use of proper-fitting equipment, loose clothing, and protective skin creams.

Head and Neck

When biking, you should always wear a protective helmet. Regrettably, when one of my patients was 15 years old, he was biking without his helmet. He collided with a car, fell to the ground, and lost consciousness for several minutes. In retrospect, he was quite lucky. At the hospital, the scans of his brain were normal, and he recovered fully. Because there was a loss of consciousness (medically known as a transient neurologic impairment), he suffered a concussion. But, he took a significant risk; he never should have been biking without a helmet. He could have been seriously hurt or even killed.

An 18-year-old helmeted hockey player from Boston University was not as fortunate. After hitting his head directly on the boards during active play, he fractured his cervical spine and suffered permanent pa-

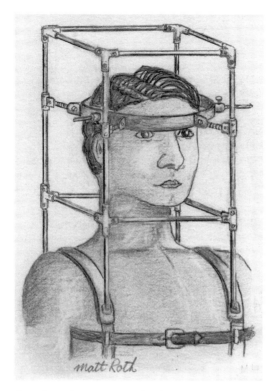

Spinal cord injuries can lead to paralysis. Wearing a helmet when biking or playing contact sports like ice hockey is a good way to prevent them. With a spinal column fracture, immobilization is necessary until the bones heal.

ralysis of his arms and legs. In hockey, it is best to remember the slogan, "HEADS UP, DON'T DUCK." (The Massachusetts Medical Society has been actively promoting this slogan.)

If you hurt your head, face, or neck while playing sports, your coach should be able to determine if you should return to the game. Coaches have guidelines that help them evaluate injuries and decide who should or should not continue to play.

A 17-year-old high school senior was accidentally hit in the face by the instructor during a self-defense class. Immediately, blood began gushing from his nose, and he was taken to the local hospital. The first round of x-rays was indecisive. A second round found that his nose had been fractured. Months later, after graduation, a surgical repair of the nose was performed.

Because of its prominence, the nose is the face's most common fracture site. In some sports, such as football, helmets give some head and face protection; in other sports, however, such as basketball, noses are quite vulnerable and may be easily broken.

If you suffer a black eye—a contusion or bruise in the skin around the eye—you should have it evaluated to rule out a fracture to the surrounding bones or a direct injury to the eyeball. Protective eye gear is important for cyclists who need to guard against flying objects, insects, and dust, and for baseball batters, hockey players, and those who participate in racquet sports such as tennis, racquetball, and squash. It might also be a good idea to wear protective eye gear if you participate in large ball sports.

I once saw an 18-year-old scuba diver for an earache. Upon examination, I discovered that his eardrum was ruptured, a condition known as barotitis media. When I questioned him, he told me that he had taken a deep dive while he had a cold. Water pressure had caused his eardrum to rupture. You should not scuba dive if you have any upper respiratory illness, it may very well trigger problems in the middle ear.

It is not uncommon for boxers and wrestlers to suffer earlobe injuries. Direct injury may result in hemorrhaging or bleeding. Repeated injuries may cause the earlobes to take on a cauliflower-like appearance. Be sure to wear the prescribed headgear.

A 16-year-old adolescent was playing street hockey when he was hit in the mouth by a hockey stick. Half of his front tooth was found on the ground. Using artificial materials, his dentist was able to fix his broken tooth, and it now looks "natural." But there is no guarantee how it will fare in the future. Sometimes, the nerves die and a dentist must perform a root canal. It might be necessary to cover the tooth with a crown. Crowns may be quite costly. During hockey, it is best to wear a mouth guard—as this adolescent now does. Typically, mouth guards are horseshoe-shaped pieces of plastic that are worn in the mouth. Mouth guards protect the teeth by blunting the impact of a potentially injurious force. They are used in other sports such as football, ice hockey, and basketball as well.

Chest

A 15-year-old patient came to see me after a collision during football practice. He had chest pain with tenderness over several of his ribs. X-rays showed that some of the ribs had hairline fractures. He was given a rib support and pain relievers. Thankfully, most chest injuries are not serious—though they may be quite painful. Be certain that you wear all the required protective gear.

Abdomen

One of my patients, an 18-year-old who was preparing to enter a military academy, became ill with a sore throat and fatigue. Unaware that he had mononucleosis, he continued his regular exercise program, which included daily calisthenics. One day, while he was completing his calisthenics routines, he felt faint and lost consciousness. Rushed to the hospital, physicians determined that his spleen had ruptured and was bleeding into his abdominal cavity. Mononucleosis had made the spleen swollen and prone to injury. Thanks to prompt medical care, he recovered and entered the military academy on schedule. While it is unusual for the spleen to rupture during sports, if you are not feeling well, you should seek medical attention before continuing your sports activities. If there is a risk that you will be struck by propelled objects—as catchers and goalies might—it is important for you to wear protective gear.

Genitourinary

Cycling outside on a beautiful day sounds like a wonderful form of exercise. But the saddle of the bike may cause bleeding in the urine due to repeated bumping action in the groin. And injury to the testicles in the form of a contusion or bruise may occur during contact and collision sports. In these sports, one should consider the use of a hard cup. Bleeding into the urine may also occur after long-distance running or horseback riding.

Bones, Ligaments, Tendons, and Joints

Shoulder Injuries

As a pole vaulter was coming down from his jump, he landed on his extended right arm. He immediately experienced shooting pain in his right shoulder. X-rays showed no fracture, but his upper arm bone (the humerus) was dislocated from the shoulder joint. A physician used manual manipulation to put the shoulder back into its joint. After the shoulder is manipulated into place in such a case, it is usually immobilized for several weeks by either a sling or brace to promote healing of the injured tissues. After the immobilization period, rehabilitation is initiated, followed by a muscle-strengthening program. The pain associated with a dislocation is treated either by nonsteroidal analgesics, such as ibuprofen, or by narcotics.

Sports-related shoulder injuries are less common than knee injuries. When they do occur, they most often affect the muscle and supporting structures such as ligaments and tendons. Around your shoulder, the back muscles hold the joint tighter than the front muscles. That is why dislocations are more commonly seen in the front. Occasionally, an athlete will describe how his arm popped forward and then snapped back. The snapping back is known as subluxation. Once the bone is back in place, it should be immobilized for several weeks. If an athlete has recurrent dislocations of his shoulder, then surgical repair may be indicated.

The rotator cuff refers to the series of muscles, tendons, and supporting structures that figure in shoulder function. Injuries to the rotator cuff are seen in sports such as baseball (especially in pitchers), swimming, and football, where repetitive overhead arm motion is common. The overuse of the rotator cuff may result in inflammation, pain, and limited motion, and the symptoms worsen with repeated overhead motion. Treatment includes rest, anti-inflammatory medications (such as ibuprofen and naprosyn), and strengthening exercises.

Fractures of the clavicle—the bone connecting the sternum to the shoulder joint—are generally not serious. Commonly seen in football and wrestling, these are treated for several weeks, either with a sling or a "figure of eight" bandage, which loops around the armpits and neck creating an X configuration on the chest and back.

Elbow

A 15-year-old patient came to see me for pain in his pitching arm, which began the previous evening during a game. X-rays were negative, and he was diagnosed with "Little League elbow."

In adolescents who have not yet completed their growth, the pitching action may cause increased traction. Little League elbow is typically a result of a traction, or pulling injury, to a knob called the medial epicondyle on the lower part of the upper arm bone (humerus). Generally, rest and anti-inflammatory medications provide relief. If you suffer from Little League elbow, you should make a gradual return to sports. In order to reduce the incidence and severity of such an injury, Little League regulations usually limit the amount of pitching by each player. For example, a 15–16-year-old player may have a limit of 107 pitches per game and no more than 2.5 games per week.

The elbow joint is a bit complicated; a number of muscles enable you to flex and extend your arm. Still other muscles allow you to turn your palm forward and backward. Tennis elbow usually occurs following overuse (working too long) and overload (working too hard); it is commonly seen in tennis players who are not preconditioned. Elbow pain occurs in the knob called the lateral epicondyle. If you are standing with your arms at your sides and your palms turned to the front, the lateral epicondyle may be felt on the inside of the elbow. In tennis elbow, the pain comes from an inflammation of the supporting tissues. Treatment

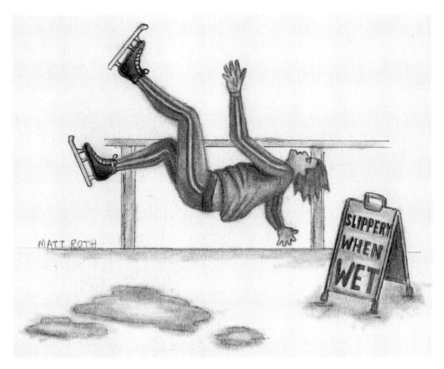

Slipping and landing on an outstretched hand can cause fractures of the lower arm.

includes rest, anti-inflammatory medications, and rehabilitation. Athletes may help prevent tennis elbow by limiting their time on the court—especially early in the season. As in many sports, overuse injuries are more likely to occur early in the season, when the muscles are not adequately conditioned.

Lower Arm

A 17-year-old cross-country runner tripped over a tree root and landed on his outstretched hand. Immediately, he had pain in his wrist. X-rays showed a chip fracture of the end of his radius (one of the lower arm bones). His arm was placed in a cast for four weeks and he has since done well, although he still has some pain during wet weather. These fractures are common in long-distance runners.

Wrist

An 18-year-old basketball player came to see me for two lingering problems. He had mild discomfort of his right wrist, and he could not

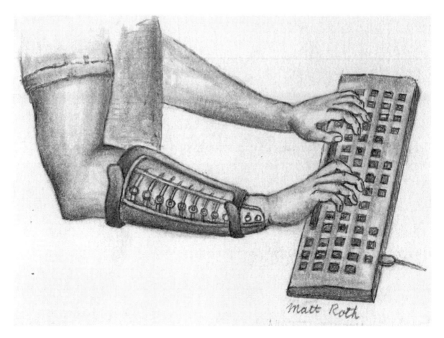

Repetitive wrist motion may lead to a fairly common condition, known as carpal tunnel syndrome. Treatment may include rest, anti-inflammatory medications, splints, and rehabilitation.

move his right wrist as well as he moved his left. X-rays showed an old fracture of a wrist bone (the scaphoid). My patient remembered that several months earlier he had fallen on his outstretched right hand during a basketball game. At first, his wrist hurt. But since it appeared to improve, he forgot about the incident. The fractured bone had not healed, and he required a surgical repair with a bone graft. A piece of bone was transplanted from his hip to the wrist to begin the healing process.

The wrist is a small but complicated part of the body. It has a number of bones, ligaments, and tendons, and it is relatively easily injured or overused. The lower arm bones (the radius and ulna) are connected to the eight carpal (wrist) bones; these, in turn, are connected to the five metacarpals (bones in the hands that connect the fingers to the wrists) and the 14 phalanges or finger bones. To reduce the risk of injury to your wrists, especially in certain sports such as skating, you may wish to use wrist guards. You should know, however, that the research findings are not conclusive. While some researchers believe that people who wear wrist guards are less likely to suffer fractures, and that the fractures that they do sustain are less serious, others contend that wrist guards are of little value. I would tend to favor them, and I encourage my patients to wear them.

Repetitive wrist motion may lead to a fairly common condition known as carpal tunnel syndrome. In this syndrome, the nerves passing through the connective tissue of the wrist are compressed, causing pain and numbness in the fingers, wrists, hands, and sometimes the upper arms. Adolescents who keyboard a great deal may already be familiar with this problem. It is also prevalent among wheelchair athletes, pitchers, and tennis players. Treatment begins by determining the cause of the problem. Then rest, anti-inflammatory medications, splints, and rehabilitation may be indicated.

Hand and Finger

Frustrated with his inability to understand his calculus assignment, a 17-year-old football player took out his anger on his bedroom wall with a powerful punch. The wall was smashed, and my patient fractured two metacarpals (the bones that end with your knuckles). The bones had to be set, and my patient wore a cast for several weeks. His days of hitting the wall are over. This type of injury is known as boxer's fracture.

As he was desperately trying to catch a pass, an 18-year-old baseball player fully extended his hand. The ball hit his second finger hard. Within moments, the player felt pain in his second finger. X-rays revealed a chip fracture in the joint. The recommended treatment was a splint.

Finger injuries most frequently occur in collision sports, such as football, and sports in which players need to catch a ball, such as basketball and baseball. Of course, it is also possible to fracture a finger in any fall, whether during a ski run or in gymnastics training.

Thigh and Hip

Most injuries to the thigh and hip affect the muscles or supporting structures. The muscles in the front of the thigh are called the quadriceps; those in the back are the hamstrings; those on the inside are the adductors. At least 16 different muscles enable the thigh to move.

A 14-year-old place kicker missed the ball during a kicking action and developed immediate pain in the front of his thigh. Excessive contraction injured his thigh muscles, and a diagnosis of quadriceps strain was made. Treatment includes RICE (rest, ice, compression, and elevation). Rehabilitation and a gradual return to sports is indicated. Quadriceps injuries are most common in soccer, rugby, and football.

The hamstring muscles, located on the back of the thigh, are commonly injured or reinjured. Runners and sprinters, who suddenly stretch their muscles, are particularly prone to this type of injury. The athlete develops pain in the muscle itself. Once again, the treatment is RICE, anti-inflammatory medications, and a slow return to sports.

Ice hockey and football players, as well as high jumpers, are susceptible to groin or adductor strains. Overstretching or a forceful contraction
of the thigh adductors, located on the inside of the thighs, may cause
injury and pain. Since the adductor muscles attach the femur to the pel-
vis, pain from overstretching of these muscles may occur in the groin
and thigh. Treatment is the same as for other muscles strains—RICE and
rehabilitation.

Knee

To better understand knee injuries, we should begin with a brief an-
atomical description of the knee. There are four major bones in the region
of the knee—the femur or thigh bone, the patella or knee cap, and the
lower leg bones known as the tibia, or shin bone, and the fibula. The
femur is connected to the tibia through the knee, which is a hinge-like
joint. Ligaments help to keep the femur, patella, tibia, and fibula in align-
ment. Between the femur and the tibia are cushion-like pads of tissue
called menisci. Ligaments and menisci are prone to injury during sports.

At the beginning of the chapter, we mentioned a football player who
suffered a torn meniscus from a clipping injury. Severe twisting of the
tibia causes the stretching of the medial collateral ligament, which, in
turn, may rupture the medial meniscus. A sharp pain will be felt over
the knee joint. If the meniscus is also torn, it may need to be repaired or
excised. A course of rehabilitation is then usually recommended.

The anterior cruciate ligament is strong tissue, which connects the femur to the tibia and helps to stabilize the knee joint. Injuries to this
ligament may occur when a sudden directional change places a strong
force on it. The ligament may tear or rupture; there is a popping sound
following by pain and the sensation of an unstable joint. Expect consid-
erable swelling. Sometimes rehabilitation and strengthening exercises are
unable to correct the problem; in that case, surgical reconstruction may
be necessary.

There are three other important knee problems that affect athletes.
Patellofemoral syndrome is a disorder in which the patella does not
move in a normal manner during flexion and extension of the knee.
Characterized by knee pain, it is best treated with conditioning, quadriceps strengthening, and precompetition stretching.

In Osgood-Schlatter disease, which is seen in growing adolescents,
there is pain below the knee cap. The pain, which usually occurs during
exercise, is caused by pulling of the tendon connecting the knee cap to
the tibia. It is aggravated by activities such as running and stepping, and
it is helped by rest. The patellar tendon itself may become inflamed and
cause patellar tendinitis (inflammation of the tendon) or jumper's knee.
This is regularly seen in players of jumping sports, such as volleyball
and basketball. The inflamed tendon is best treated with rest, anti-
inflammatory medications, and rehabilitation.

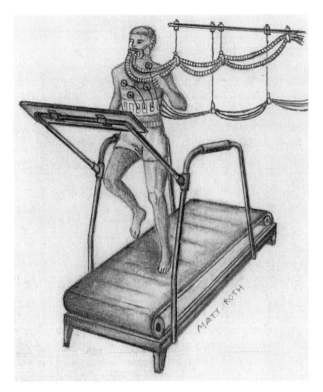

Reconditioning exercises may be necessary after some sport injuries.

A thirteen year old came to me with a one-day history of pain in his right knee. An x-ray showed osteochondritis dissecans which occurs when a portion of the bone separates from the end of the femur. The cartilage, which is fibrous connective tissue around the bone fragment and feels like the tip of your nose, may stay intact and hold the bone fragment next to the bone. Or, the cartilage may separate from the piece of bone and float in the knee joint. Symptoms include knee pain, locking of the knee, poor function, or an unstable knee joint and swelling. Treatment may include rest, casting, and/or arthroscopic removal of the loose body of the bone. The arthroscope is an instrument that allows a small incision to be made through which a camera and small instruments enable the surgeon to perform the surgery.

Leg

A 15-year-old long-distance runner came to me early in the season for lower leg pain. The discomfort was particularly intense at the end of a run along rural country roads. He was found to have shin splints, or pain along the front of the legs between the top of the tibia and the ankle. Shin splints are believed to be caused by inflammation of the tissue covering the bone. Typically, they are seen early in the season in poorly conditioned runners who are running on hard pavement such as asphalt. Warming up, running on softer surfaces, good running shoes, anti-inflammatory drugs, and strengthening exercises may help.

Another overuse syndrome of the leg is achilles tendinitis. In this disorder the achilles tendon, which connects the calf muscle (gastrocnemius) to the heel, is inflamed. Athletes describe local tenderness, usually near the heel. Sudden intense training, poor footwear, running on hard surfaces, and overuse may be contributing factors. In addition to rest, anti-inflammatory medications, rehabilitation, and orthotics may be useful.

Ankle

The most common sports injury is the sprained ankle. Ankle injuries comprise up to 45 percent of all basketball injuries and about 25 percent of all injuries in volleyball.

The ankle consists of two joints with three bones. One joint allows the foot to move up and down, the other permits the foot to turn inward and outward and to rotate. Ligaments of soft tissue connect these bones and provide stability. A sprain occurs when abnormal movement or force causes these ligaments to be stretched or torn. About 85 percent of sprains happen when the foot twists on its outer side (an inversion injury), producing force on the outside ligaments. There is pain and swelling and sometimes bruising of the outside of the ankle. Treatment consists of an ankle brace and RICE. Sprains are graded from 1 to 3. The more severe sprains may require splinting or surgery. Return to play may vary from one to ten days for a grade 1 sprain to up to two months for a grade 3 sprain.

Foot

After walking ten miles for the Walk for Hunger in poorly fitted shoes, a 20-year-old patient came to see me for pain in his heel. The area where the achilles tendon attached to the heel was inflamed, a condition known as apophysitis of the calcaneus (heel). An x-ray revealed some bone irregularity in the area. This condition is often seen in the landing foot for lay-ups in basketball. Anti-inflammatory drugs, rest, and proper fitting shoes are useful treatments.

On occasion, a teen will come to see me with pain and tenderness in the arch of the foot. This problem, which is seen in long-distance runners, especially those running on hills, and in athletes who wear ill-fitting shoes, is called plantar fasciitis. In this case, the fascia, or the fibrous tissue below the skin, has become inflamed, strained, or torn. Treatment consists of proper footwear, rehabilitation, anti-inflammatory medication, and taping.

A hyperextension or twisting upward of the great toe may cause turf toe in runners and those who play on artificial turf. Damage to the soft tissue in the toe causes pain and swelling. Treatment includes RICE and anti-inflammatory medications.

Although they might appear to be strong, toenails are actually quite prone to injury, especially when the athlete does not wear shoes. Of all the toenails, the great toenail is the most vulnerable. Taping the nail may offer some protection. But blood may still form under the toenail, a condition known as subungual hematoma, particularly when playing a sport like soccer or tennis. The average soccer player loses two or three toenails (that grow back) a year from such blood formations. Treatment includes penetrating the nail with a hot clip or drill to allow the blood to drain.

Pain in the ball of the foot is known as metatarsalgia. This is seen in runners who run on their toes. Putting soft inlays in shoes may be helpful in alleviating this condition.

Back

One of my patients, a 16-year-old gymnast, came to my office with low back pain. He told me that during his routines he would hyperextend his back. Over time, these movements caused a series of small injuries (microtrauma) to the low back. Eventually, those injuries created a lesion or spondylolysis in the vertebra. Usually the back pain is on one side and is worsened by hyperextending the back. Rest is the best treatment for spondylolysis. You should be aware that many of these conditions are uncommon, and most are easily cured.

SPORTS MEDICINE

While everyone agrees that exercise is an integral part of a healthy lifestyle, sometimes participation in sports may have negative health consequences. Should you exercise when you are sick? This is a difficult question to answer, but here are some general guidelines:

- If you have a mild illness, such as a cold, but do not have a fever, light exercise is okay.
- If exercising while ill makes you feel worse, then discontinue exercise until you feel better.
- If you have an illness that requires medical attention, ask your medical provider when you can resume exercising. You may also wish to ask what type of exercise would be appropriate.
- You should realize that, when you are ill, some of your body's energy is focused on the symptoms of the illness (such as coughing) or on fighting the infection. Thus, your level of performance may be diminished.
- Medications used in treatment of the illness may affect performance.

Now let's review each body system for particular sports-related problems.

Skin

Athlete's foot, or tinea pedis, is a fungal infection that grows best in warm, moist, and dark areas of the body. That is why the foot and spaces between the toes are especially prone to this infection. Athlete's foot causes the skin to be itchy, red, and scaly. One of the best places to catch athlete's foot is on the locker room floor. Always wear shoes or clogs when walking around a locker room. Athlete's foot is treated with antifungal creams, such as Spectazole or Lotrimin, cotton socks to prevent perspiration, and frequent bathing.

During baseball season, an 18-year-old patient came to see me because of red, itchy, hot areas around his scrotum and inner thighs. He had a disease called jock itch, or tinea cruris, which is caused by a fungus that thrives in the genital region. Treatment includes an antifungal cream, frequent changes of cotton underwear, and at least one daily shower. Excessive perspiration tends to promote fungal growth.

The herpes simplex skin infection may be transmitted during skin-to-skin contact, such as in wrestling, or even from virus deposits on wrestling equipment. Wrestling mats should be scrubbed after each practice or competition. Herpes transmission may also occur in other contact sports, such as basketball. Upon infection, patients develop a painful rash of blisters, which eventually break and then scab over. Treatment may include an antiviral medication, such as acyclovir, and, occasionally, pain relievers.

Bacteria such as staph or strep may cause painful skin infections such as impetigo. These may be acquired during contact sports. Symptoms include a red, honeycombed rash with blisters. The infection is treated with topical antibiotics such as bacitracin or bactroban.

Wart viruses may trigger the growth of plantar warts on the bottom of the feet. Plantar warts are hard and uncomfortable. You can easily get them by walking barefoot on a surface where someone with an active wart has recently walked. Plantar warts should be frozen with liquid nitrogen.

Lungs

At the beginning of this chapter, we described a cross-country runner who developed problems with breathing during the biggest race of the season. He was diagnosed with exercise-induced asthma (EIA). EIA more often occurs in cold and dry weather and in certain sports such as cross country, ice skating, and soccer. It is believed to be related to the duration and level of exercise. Since a high rate of respiration dries and cools the airway, a higher level of exertion could cause the body to narrow the bronchi (bronchospasm). Interestingly, it is rare for swimmers to suffer from EIA. But their environment is obviously warmer and moister.

EIA will cause progressive shortness of breath and wheezing. Teens with EIA should seek medical assistance. An exercise challenge test may be ordered. There are good treatment regimens, including inhalers such as bronchodilators, anti-inflammatory agents, or allergy cell stabilizers, which prevent the body from releasing EIA-triggering substances. Usually, the best treatment is to inhale a bronchodilator 15 to 30 minutes before the beginning of competition.

Intestines

It is not uncommon for runners to suffer from runner's diarrhea. This problem begins with cramps and the urge to have a bowel movement. That is followed by diarrhea. No one is certain exactly what causes this problem. Some say that athletes tend to eat diets that are high in bulk, which bring on abdominal cramps. Others maintain that the diarrhea stems from precompetition nervousness. Ordinarily, the diarrhea is not severe enough to cause serious concern. However, to prevent dehydration, it is important to maintain your fluid balance. If you have diarrhea, be sure to continue drinking water or a balanced electrolyte solution.

Some athletes also experience gastroesophageal reflux disease (GERD), in which the stomach contents are released back into the esophagus, causing pain and heartburn. This may be due to a malfunctioning valve between the esophagus and the stomach. This allows the stomach contents to push back up into the esophagus. Treatment strategies include avoiding caffeine, elevating the head of the bed, refraining from large meals within three hours of bedtime, taking antacids, and taking medications prescribed by your medical provider.

Ears

Scuba diving may cause a variety of ear problems. For each 32 feet of descent, the water pressure increases by one atmosphere. One atmosphere is the pressure of air on an individual at sea level. Therefore, at two atmospheres, the pressure is doubled. This pressure may cause injuries outlined in Chapter 9, on outdoor and wilderness health. Also, it may cause hearing loss, ringing in the ears, or vertigo.

Exercising or competing in environments with loud noises may lead to hearing loss. Reports of hearing loss have occurred after exposure to noise levels of 85 decibels (a level noted at loud rock concerts) over eight hours. Obviously, it is best to prevent exposure to such loud noises.

Kidneys

After the Boston Marathon, a long-distance runner came to see me complaining about discolored urine. His red urine was found to contain blood. This is known as traumatic hematuria (blood in the urine) and it is fairly common in long-distance runners and swimmers. It happens for one of two reasons: Either the nephrons—urine-filtration units in the kidneys—release blood into the urine, or areas in the bladder bleed. While these events sound ominous, they are normally benign. A cyclist may also find blood in his urine from bumps to his perineum (area between the anus and scrotum), which may be caused by rough roads. Tilting the nose of the bike seat downward may help prevent such bleeding in the urine. Still, blood in the urine should be evaluated by a physician to rule out more serious causes. And any direct injury to the kidneys, which could cause permanent damage, should always be examined by a physician.

Hormones

Adolescents who have diabetes mellitus do not produce a sufficient amount of insulin, a hormone, to properly regulate their blood sugar. As a result, they take measured amounts of insulin by injection to control the amount of sugar in their bloodstream. Because prolonged exercise encourages sugar to enter the cells and leave the bloodstream, an adolescent with diabetes may develop hypoglycemia or low blood sugar. Thus, a diabetic may need to adjust his insulin downward prior to exercise or eat a snack. The symptoms of hypoglycemia include sweating, nervousness, shaking, and hunger. A sugar snack will stop the symptoms.

Blood

Sports anemia should not be confused with true anemia. It should more appropriately be called a pseudoanemia. In this condition, the adolescent's level of hemoglobin (the red pigment in blood cells that carries oxygen) is slightly below normal. It is believed to be caused by the dilution of the bloodstream with fluid, thereby increasing the volume of the teen's blood. This is thought to be the body's adaptation to endurance training and has no effect on athletic competitiveness.

Muscles

In order to lose weight, a college freshman decided to begin an exercise program. On the first day, he did 100 sit-ups. The next day, he was at my office complaining of soreness in his abdomen. Delayed Onset Muscle Soreness is caused by the overuse of muscles in poorly conditioned people. The muscles become sore and swollen, but slowly return to normal. A gradual exercise program is the best preventive measure.

Emotions

Runner's high is found in well-conditioned, long-distance runners. Described as a euphoria, or state of general relaxation, it is thought to be due to the release of endorphins into the body. Endorphins are naturally produced substances that elevate your mood and alleviate pain.

"Exercise addiction" is more common than most people realize. Although addiction is probably too strong a term, some athletes who experience "runner's highs" may become dependent on exercise for mood elevation. Without exercise, these athletes develop a negative mood or depression. If an adolescent reaches a point where he neglects other life activities—including studies, work, friends, or family—in favor of exercising compulsively, this has the potential to become a serious problem.

Neurologic

A 19-year-old weight lifter came to me for headaches that were precipitated by his weight-lifting routines. Typically, these headaches were centered in the back of his head and continued for several days. Known as "weight-lifter's headaches," these type of headaches are probably due to strained ligaments in the neck.

Athletes may suffer from other types of sports-related headaches. Benign exertional headache is brief in duration and related to activity. Acute-effort migraine may develop after a short period of intensive exercise. Unlike the benign exertional headache, the athlete may have visual disturbances, nausea, and vomiting. Persistent or frequent headaches should be evaluated by a physician.

REFERENCES

Churchill, R. S., and B. G. Donley. "Managing Injuries of the Great Toe." *The Physician and Sportsmedicine* 26 (September 1998) 9: 29–39.

Committee on Injury and Poison Prevention. *Injury Prevention and Control for Children and Youth, 3rd Edition*. Elk Grove Village, Ill.: American Academy of Pediatrics, 1997.

Committee on Sports Medicine and Fitness. *Sports Medicine: Health Care for Young Athletes, 2nd Edition*. Elk Grove Village, Ill.: American Academy of Pediatrics, 1991.

Fields, Karl B., and Peter A. Fricker, editors. *Medical Problems in Athletes*. Oxford, England: Blackwell Science, 1997.

Greydanus, Donald E., Dilip R. Patel, and Euguene F. Luckstead, editors. *Office Orthopedics and Sports Medicine, Adolescent Medicine: State of the Art Reviews*. Philadelphia: Hanley & Belfus, Inc., 1998.

Hergenroeder, Albert C., and James G. Garrick, editors. *Sports Medicine, The Pediatrics Clinics of North America*. Philadelphia: W. B. Saunders Co., 1990.

Mellion, Morris B., editor. *Office Sports Medicine, 2nd Edition*. Philadelphia: Henley & Belfus, Inc., 1996.

Pappas, Arthur M., editor. *Upper Extremity Injuries in the Athlete*. New York: Churchill Livingstone Inc., 1995.

Post, W. R. "Patellofemoral Pain." *The Physician and Sportsmedicine* 26 (January 1998) 1: 68–78.

Tanzi, E., and R. Scher. "Managing Common Nail Disorders in Active Patients and Athletes." *The Physician and Sportsmedicine* 27 (September 1999) 9: 35–47.

Trojian, T. H., and D. B. McKeag. "Ankle Sprains." *The Physician and Sportsmedicine* 26 (October 1998) 10: 29–40.

Vinger, Paul F., and Earl F. Hoerner, editors. *Sports Injuries, 2nd Edition*. Littleton, Mass.: PSG Publishing Co., Inc., 1986.

Wall, E. J. "Osgood-Schlatter Disease." *The Physician and Sportsmedicine* 26 (March 1998) 3: 29–34.

Wang, T. W., W. D. Knopp, C. A. Bush-Joseph, and B. R. Bach. "Osteochrondritis Dissecans of the Knee." *The Physician and Sportsmedicine* 26 (August 1998) 8: 31–36.

Whiteside, J. A., J. R. Andrews, and G. S. Fleisig. "Elbow Injuries in Young Baseball Players." *The Physician and Sportsmedicine* 27 (June 1999) 6: 87–102.

8

Adolescent Medical Concerns and Practices

ACNE

Acne is a skin condition seen in 85 percent of adolescents. It is caused by sex hormones that trigger an increased production of a substance called sebum from glands found in your face, upper back, and chest. The higher amounts of sebum plug your skin follicles. There is also more growth of a specific bacteria that leads to acne. Here are some facts about acne:

- Blackheads are plugged skin follicles with a black coloration.
- Papules are inflamed (often red) pimples.
- Pustules are papules with a central core of pussy, white material.

Generally, acne takes time to treat—often months. And stress may exacerbate the condition and delay improvement. Although many people contend that acne is a result of a diet that includes chocolate, nuts, and french fries, that belief has not been proven by scientific studies.

There are a number of topical treatments. For example, benzoyl peroxide kills the acne bacteria and helps dissolve the sebum plugs. Retin-A, available by prescription, decreases the plugging of the follicles. Erythromycin or clindamycin, found in topical antibiotics, help kill the acne bacteria.

But there are also oral medications. Taken orally, erythromycin, tetracycline, or minocycline decrease the amount of acne bacteria. These prescription drugs are useful for moderate acne that has not responded to topical treatment. For the most severe acne, there is accutane, a synthetic vitamin A derivative that cuts down on the growth of acne bacteria as well as sebum. While it is highly effective, it has many potentially negative side effects.

AIDS (ACQUIRED IMMUNODEFICIENCY SYNDROME)

AIDS, which is caused by the HIV virus, is contracted through the exchange of body fluids (semen, vaginal secretions, and blood) and may be transmitted by unprotected anal or vaginal intercourse, or the sharing of intravenous needles. Those at highest risk for acquiring HIV engage in unprotected anal, receptive intercourse; unprotected insertive, anal intercourse poses the next highest risk. Transmission is less likely in vaginal intercourse, but the virus has been transmitted during oral sex. Properly using latex condoms for vaginal or anal intercourse, and dental dams for oral sex, will markedly reduce the risk of transmission. Condoms are available at many stores. But dental dams may be more difficult to obtain. Some teens carefully cut a nonlatex condom (which is not bitter to taste), and use this as a barrier when performing oral sex on a female. Males should wear a condom when having oral sex performed on them. Obviously, sharing needles or going to unlicensed tattoo parlors should be avoided.

If you are worried that you may have acquired HIV, an antibody test is available. You should have the test done at a center where pre- and post-test counseling are available. Testing at these centers is usually anonymous. You will be identified by a number, not a name. Some centers will allow you to pay directly, so no bill is sent to your home. You may have heard that home testing kits for HIV are available in some states. Do not use them, as they may be inaccurate, and the counseling given to you with the test results may be incorrect and unhelpful. Confidential tests may also be done. But, your name is noted on the result, and the result will become part of your medical record. Usually confidential HIV test results are stored in a separate section of your medical record and may not be released with your other records.

Years ago, people with HIV almost always died within a few years. Now, there are effective, long-term treatments that are prolonging life indefinitely. For many people, HIV is a chronic disease, not a death sentence. But it requires specialized care. So, if there is a chance that you may test positive for HIV, it is important that you know. See Chapter 5 for more information.

ALLERGY (HAY FEVER, SEASONAL)

Allergy symptoms include runny nose, sneezing, itchy eyes, and sore throat. These may be caused by a variety of environmental factors such as grasses, flowers, trees, weeds, and animals as well as indoor agents, including dust or dust mites. Treatment includes antihistamines or nasal sprays, such as nasal steroids. The newer prescription oral antihistamines usually do not cause drowsiness.

ALOPECIA (HAIR LOSS, BALDNESS)

Baldness is usually hereditary, transmitted through the mother's genes. Some males susceptible to baldness begin to lose hair in their teens, especially around the temples. But significant baldness does not generally occur until well beyond adolescence. Topical treatment agents include nonprescription minoxidil. If you are losing your hair, you should consult a physician for evaluation and possible prescription medication.

ASTHMA

In this condition, bronchi—the tubes between the trachea (windpipe) and lungs—have an increased sensitivity to certain triggers, including allergic agents, exercise, cold air, smoke, and respiratory infections. With asthma, the bronchi constrict, which impedes the flow of exhaled air. There are a variety of treatments for asthma, including inhaled bronchodilators, anti-inflammatory agents such as inhaled steroids, and medications that curtail the allergic process. Most teens with asthma are able to participate fully in physical activities.

BALDNESS

See Alopecia.

BEDWETTING (ENURESIS)

Bedwetting may be a very stressful problem, and it tends to run in families. If both parents were bedwetters, there is a 77 percent chance that their children will wet their beds. Between 1 percent and 3 percent of adolescents between the ages of 12 and 18 wet their beds. Successful treatments include medications such as DDAVP or imipramine (Tofranil). DDAVP is a substance that temporarily limits the amount of urine produced. It is not totally understood how Tofranil works, but it is thought to make the patient more sensitive to a full bladder and awaken more readily. Bedwetters should be evaluated and followed closely by a medical professional.

BODY PIERCING

Although many parents may be troubled by body piercing, there is historical precedent for such activities. Egyptian pharaohs were known to pierce their navels, and Roman soldiers pierced their nipples. Body jewelry can be made from surgical stainless steel, titanium, gold, or niobium. Male teens have been known to pierce their eyebrows, tongues, nipples, navels, and penises. But you should be aware that many potential medical problems may be caused by body piercing. These include contracting hepatitis B and C, infection, excessive bleeding, allergic reactions, nerve damage, dental problems, and scarring. Penis piercing may damage the penis. And many females are turned off by body jewelry, especially on the penis.

CHEST PAIN

Although chest pain is a common complaint in adolescent males, the cause is rarely serious. A "stitch" is characterized as a short, sharp, and sudden pain in the chest worsened with deep breathing or bending. The cause is unknown. A chest muscle strain—either from exercise, lifting, or coughing—may cause injuries to the chest muscles with resulting pain. Inflammation of the cartilage attaching the rib to the breastbone—termed costochondritis—may also account for chest pain. However, problems with the lungs, heart, and gastrointestinal system may trigger chest pain as well, so if the pain persists, you may wish to check with your medical provider.

CHICKEN POX

Chicken pox is a common childhood illness caused by the varicella virus. It is characterized by a fever and a very itchy, bumpy body rash. During the past few years, a vaccine has become available. If you have not had chicken pox by the time you graduate from high school, you should have the vaccine.

Chicken pox in adults is a far more serious illness, and it sometimes causes potentially serious complications.

CHOLESTEROL

Cholesterol is a blood fat that plays a vital role in the body's metabolism. When your blood has an elevated amount of this substance, it may cause premature heart disease. There is no consensus among health professionals on which adolescents should be screened for elevated cholesterol, done with a simple blood test. Maintaining a balanced diet and a regular exercise program may help control your cholesterol.

CHRONIC FATIGUE SYNDROME

This is an illness in which the patient has overwhelming fatigue and a host of other symptoms, such as muscle aches, low fevers, sleep disorders, depression, and impaired thinking. Unfortunately, there is no specific test to diagnose chronic fatigue, and it may be easily misdiagnosed. There is also no known cause. A medication called Florinef, which enhances the absorption of sodium and increases the patient's blood pressure, has been helpful for some patients.

COMMON COLD

The common cold is the most frequently occurring infection in adolescent males. It is characterized by sore throat, runny nose, low fever, cough, and headache, and it usually lasts about a week. There are over 100 viruses that may cause a cold. Treatment entails relieving the discomfort with acetaminophen (Tylenol), plenty of fluids, and, occasionally, a mild decongestant or cough suppressant.

CONTACT DERMATITIS

Contact dermatitis is an itchy skin rash caused by contact with an irritating substance such as poison oak, poison ivy, or poison sumac. It is more common in the warmer months, when there is a greater amount of outside activity. Other causes of contact dermatitis include allergies to nickel, clothing dyes, adhesive tape, and rubber and/or latex compounds. Treatment includes removing or avoiding the irritating substances, topical steroid creams, antihistamines to relieve itch, and, in severe cases, the use of oral steroids.

CYSTIC FIBROSIS

Cystic fibrosis is an inherited, lifelong disorder, in which an abnormal substance is produced in the respiratory tract. This mucousy substance causes respiratory insufficiency, digestive distress, and, occasionally, diabetes mellitus. Patients with this illness are subject to lung infections and chronic respiratory failure.

DIABETES MELLITUS

Diabetes mellitus, or Type I diabetes, is an illness in which the pancreas, an organ in the abdomen, loses its ability to produce adequate amounts of insulin, a hormone that regulates blood sugar. As a result, the body is less able to regulate blood sugar and the levels of blood sugar rise. This causes increased urination, loss of calories, and weight loss, as well as long-term complications. Treatment includes careful monitoring of blood-sugar levels and frequent injections of insulin, which lowers blood-sugar levels to the normal range. Adolescents who have diabetes are able to carry on normal life functions (see Chapter 14 on chronic conditions).

DIARRHEA

Watery, frequent, and often explosive bowel movements may be caused by a variety of agents, such as infections, colitis (see Inflammatory Bowel Disease), food poisoning, milk, or wheat (or other food) intolerances, medications, and irritable bowel syndrome (IBS). If the diarrhea is caused by an infectious agent, it will usually pass in a few days. Sometimes, medical intervention will be required. If the diarrhea is caused by a food intolerance, then the appropriate dietary adjustments should be made. IBS is a functional disorder; although the intestine appears normal, its function is impaired. While IBS has no definite cause or treatment, its symptoms, which usually begin in late adolescence, increase with stress. In a small number of cases, diarrhea may be caused by an autoimmune disorder known as celiac disease. People with this disorder are unable to eat gluten (wheat, oats, rye, and barley) because it destroys the villi, or finger-like projections, of the small intestine. The body reacts against itself in autoimmune disorders, and this reaction may cause damage.

EJACULATION (BLOODY)

Teens or their partners may note reddish semen, which contains blood. Usually, no cause for bleeding is found. Occasionally, the blood may indicate a sexually transmitted disease. If the problem persists, a physician should be consulted.

ENURESIS

See Bedwetting.

EPIDIDYMITIS

Epididymitis is an inflammation of a small sac found on the upper part and back of each testicle. Pain is present, and there may be discharge from the urethra and a low-grade fever. Since epididymitis may indicate the presence of a sexually transmitted disease, a physician should be seen.

FAINTING

Fainting is a brief (typically less than one minute) loss of consciousness. Commonly, it is due to a decrease in the circulation of the blood to the brain, which may be caused by prolonged standing, dehydration, or fear of the sight of blood. Recovery is spontaneous. About 30 percent of adolescents faint at least once during their teen years. While most causes of fainting are relatively benign, occasionally fainting may stem from a serious heart or metabolic condition.

GROWING PAINS

This is not a disease, and many medical authorities discount its existence. Growing pains refer to an achiness in the upper and lower legs, often at night. No treatment is indicated.

HAIR LOSS

See Alopecia.

HEADACHE

Headaches are fairly common in people of all ages. Caused by contraction of the muscles of the neck and scalp, the most common type is the tension headache. These usually occur in the late afternoon. Headaches may also be triggered by eyestrain, illness, injury, and depression. Migraines are more intense headaches, which are characterized by a throbbing or pulsating sensation, usually on one side of the head. Vomiting is not uncommon. Migraine sufferers often note that there is a family history of the problem. They should be evaluated by a physician.

HEMATURIA (BLOOD IN THE URINE)

Bleeding in any location of the urinary track system may result in blood in the urine. The blood may be light red, deep red, or brown in color. There are many reasons for blood to appear in the urine. After exercise, participants in certain sports—such as long-distance running, swimming, rugby, crew, football, baseball, hockey, lacrosse, boxing, and cross-country skiing—are more likely to have blood in their urine. Usually, there is no need for treatment, but, if the problem persists, it should be checked by a medical provider.

HEPATITIS A

Transmitted by food or water or through oral or genital sex, hepatitis A is an infectious disease of the liver that is caused by a virus. To prevent this illness, I advise my patients who are at risk to take the two-dose hepatitis A vaccine. Individuals who plan travel in underdeveloped areas or who are gay should receive the vaccine.

HEPATITIS B

Like hepatitis A, hepatitis B is also an infection of the liver. It is spread in several ways, including unprotected sex, contaminated blood, from an infected mother (during childbirth), and from blood products or needles. A three-dose vaccine is available and should be taken by all adolescents to prevent this disease.

HEPATITIS C

This third form of hepatitis is spread by contaminated blood or the sharing of needles between drug abusers. Unfortunately, there is no vaccine for this type of hepatitis, and roughly half of those infected with hepatitis C develop chronic liver disease.

HERNIA

An inguinal hernia, a protrusion of tissue that may or may not be painful, arises from an opening in the canal that connects the scrotum with the body. In adolescents, a hernia is usually surgically repaired.

HIGH BLOOD PRESSURE

See Hypertension.

HIV

See AIDS.

HYDROCOELE

A hydrocoele is a sac of fluid that may envelop part of the testicle. Often, no intervention is necessary. But if it is large and cosmetically unsightly, it may be surgically repaired.

HYPERSOMNIA

Hypersomnia is excess daytime sleepiness. Most adolescent males require nine to ten hours of sleep each night. If you do not get sufficient sleep, you will have difficulty staying awake in school and while driving. Narcolepsy is a related disorder, in which people suddenly fall asleep during normal daily activities. Another sleep disorder, called sleep apnea, is caused by an obstruction of the respiratory tract that leads to frequent nighttime awakenings. Specialized sleep clinics diagnose and treat these conditions.

HYPERTENSION

Hypertension, or high blood pressure, is defined as the elevation of the blood pressure to two standard deviations or more above the average. Thus, an average blood pressure for a 16–18-year-old male would be about 118/68. So a blood pressure reading of 142/92 would be considered high. Even though there may be no symptoms, high blood pressure should be evaluated, and, possibly, treated.

HYPERTHYROIDISM

Hyperthyroidism is increased activity of the thyroid leading to excess production of the thyroid hormone. Symptoms include weight loss, wakefulness, emotional instability, and a change in school performance. Hyperthyroidism is treated with medications.

HYPOTHYROIDISM

Hypothyroidism occurs when there is a decrease in the activity of the thyroid, leading to a less than normal production of the thyroid hormone. Symptoms may include fatigue, weight gain, and decreased memory. Hypothyroidism is treated with thyroid supplements.

IMPETIGO

Impetigo is a skin infection caused by staph or strep bacteria. It is characterized by a yellow rash with a honeycomb appearance. Impetigo is treated with topical or oral antibiotics.

IMPOTENCE

This is the inability to have or to sustain an erection for sexual intercourse. For adolescents, this is typically not a hormonal or physical problem. Rather, it is usually due to psychological or emotional issues. Teens with impotence problems should consult a physician.

INFLAMMATORY BOWEL DISEASE

Inflammatory bowel disease refers to a number of gastrointestinal disorders of unknown cause, such as Crohn's disease and ulcerative colitis, which are characterized by an inflammation of some part of the intestines, rectum, or anus. The symptoms include diarrhea, which is often bloody or mucousy, and intense pain. The condition may be aggravated by stress. A physician should be consulted.

INSOMNIA

Insomnia—problems falling asleep, staying asleep, and awakening too early—are not infrequent occurrences in adolescence. Stress, caffeine, depression, or substance abuse may be contributing factors.

JOCK ITCH

Jock itch is a groin rash that often occurs during the warmer months. Caused by a fungus, it is generally red and scaly, and it appears on the upper inner thighs. Jock itch is easily treated with topical antifungal medications.

KYPHOSIS

Kyphosis is a forward curve of the upper spine which may lead to "round shoulders" and poor posture. It is generally treated with physical therapy and exercises to improve muscle tone. Surgery or braces are rarely used.

LORDOSIS

Lordosis is a backward curve of the lower spine that gives rise to "sway back." In some cases, it may be treated with a brace or surgery.

LYME DISEASE

Lyme disease, an infection caused by the spirochete Borrelia burgdorferi, is transmitted by a bite from a deer tick. Symptoms include a characteristic bull's eye rash, which occurs three to 30 days after the tick bite. Diagnosed infections are treated with antibiotics. In recent years, a three-injection vaccine series has become available for individuals 15 years of age and older. But it does not prevent all cases of symptomatic Lyme disease. The best prevention is to use tick repellent and to conduct a complete tick check after possible exposure. When working or playing in a tick-infested area, wear long sleeves and long pants with the cuffs tucked into your socks.

MASTURBATION

Masturbation refers to the self-stimulation of the penis. It is a normal activity performed by virtually 100 percent of adolescent males.

MELANOMA

Melanoma is a type of skin cancer that may first appear during the teenage years. If it is treated early, it is curable. Be alert for a mole, about the size of a pencil eraser or larger, that has different colors, bleeds, and has irregular borders or is not symmetric in appearance. Since melanoma may also appear on your back, you should ask a parent to check that area. If you are concerned about any mole, have it checked by a physician.

MENINGITIS

Meningitis is an inflammation of the covering of the brain. It is a serious infection most commonly caused by an infectious agent such as bacteria or a virus. The treatment will depend on what is causing the infection. Patients will often be hospitalized for tests and treatment.

MENINGOCOCCAL DISEASE

Meningococcal disease is a rare but serious bacterial infection that may affect teens, especially those who live in close quarters, such as dormitories. The bacteria may cause bleeding under the skin, shock, and meningitis. There is a vaccine to prevent this infection. You may wish to discuss with your medical provider if you should receive this vaccine, especially before you leave for college.

MIGRAINE

See Headache.

MONONUCLEOSIS

Mononucleosis, or mono, is an infectious disease caused by the Epstein-Barr virus. Common in adolescents, it is transmitted by kissing or other contact with oral secretions. The illness is characterized by excessive fatigue, sore throat, swollen glands, a low-grade fever, loss of appetite, and nausea. While there is no specific treatment, depending on the patient's symptoms, pain relievers and oral steroids may be prescribed. Rest is vitally important, and athletics is usually restricted for several weeks.

MORNING AFTER PILL

After at-risk sex (no condom, broken condom), a female may be prescribed an oral contraceptive to prevent pregnancy—generally referred to as the "morning after pill" or emergency contraception. If the medication is taken within 72 hours after intercourse, there is a greater than 98 percent chance that no pregnancy will occur. A healthcare provider should be consulted as soon as possible if your partner needs emergency contraception.

ORCHITIS

Orchitis is the painful inflammation of one or both testicles, which is usually due to an infection. Before the mumps vaccine was available, it was not uncommon for males to develop orchitis when they had mumps. Sometimes, this led to sterility. Fortunately, the mumps vaccine has been highly successful in preventing mumps.

PHIMOSIS

Phimosis is the inability to fully retract the foreskin in uncircumcised males. It may lead to infection or pain during intercourse. Treatment includes a surgical loosening of the foreskin or circumcision.

PINK PEARLY PENILE PAPULES

After puberty, pink pearly penile papules are harmless penile bumps that are seen in about 19 percent of males. Found on the head of the penis, where it meets the penile shaft, they are not contagious and require no treatment and they are not a sexually transmitted disease.

PLANTAR WART

A plantar wart is a growth on the bottom of a foot. Caused by a virus, it is usually passed from person to person by walking barefoot on surfaces where the virus resides. The wart can be treated with liquid nitrogen.

POSTURE

Your posture, or how you stand, may be affected by kyphosis, lordosis, or scoliosis. (See the descriptions of these terms.) Treatment may be available.

PREPARTICIPATION SPORTS EXAMINATION

This annual exam, which is highly recommended for adolescents who participate in sports, has several objectives. First, it identifies conditions that might disqualify a teen from participating in a certain sport. But it is also useful to diagnose treatable conditions and to develop treatment or rehabilitation plans for disease, injuries, or muscular-skeletal problems. Many physicians combine this exam with an annual comprehensive medical exam, which also reviews growth and development, risky behaviors, school achievement, mental health, immunizations, and other important issues.

PREVENTIVE CARE

The American Medical Association has developed annual preventive visit recommendations for adolescents. These are known as the Guidelines for Adolescent Preventive Services, or GAPS. These recommendations cover five major areas:

1. Health guidance development, diet, and healthy lifestyle
2. Screening history: sexual activity, tobacco, and alcohol use
3. Physical assessment: physical examination
4. Tests variable, but may include TB test or cholesterol screening
5. Immunizations variable, may include vaccines for hepatitis B and chicken pox

PROSTATITIS

Prostatitis is an infection of the prostate, an organ near the bladder that makes a fluid component of semen. Symptoms include pain in the bladder region, pain during ejaculation, and/or a fever. The infection may be due to a sexually transmitted disease such as gonorrhea or chlamydia.

REPETITIVE STRAIN INJURY

Persistent muscle aches, tendon inflammation, or nerve compression may develop from repeated tasks such as computer keyboarding or using a computer mouse. Constant, repetitive activity may damage tissues in your wrists and hands. Take care to ensure that your typing technique does not cause undue injury to your fingers and wrists. Be sure your wrists do not angle forward, back, or side to side. Press the keys lightly with your fingers. If you have persistent pain, see a medical provider.

SCOLIOSIS

Scoliosis is a lateral (side to side) curve of the spine that may give rise to posture problems. In most cases, there is no identifiable cause although some boys may be born with this condition. A physician should be consulted, and treatment is available if the curve is significant.

SICKLE CELL DISEASE

Sickle Cell disease is an inherited disorder in which the normal blood hemoglobin (AA), the substance in your blood that gives it the red color and carries oxygen, is replaced with sickle hemoglobin (SS). SS hemoglobin, a lifelong problem, leads to significant anemia and recurrent medical problems. People with sickle-trait hemoglobin (AS) are carriers of the disorder. While they do not have symptoms, they may pass along the trait to their children.

SLEEPWALKING

A significant minority of adolescents have at least one episode of sleepwalking. Generally, these are benign. The teen will sleepwalk for one to 30 minutes and have no memory of the experience.

SPERMATOCOELE

This is a painless cyst-like bubble in the epididymis, a sac at the top and back of each testicle, which is harmless and requires no treatment.

STREP THROAT

An infection of the throat caused by the streptococcal bacterium, strep throat is easily treated with penicillin or another antibiotic.

TATTOO

You may acquire an infection, such as hepatitis B, by going to an unlicensed tattoo parlor. Although physicians are now having some success using lasers to remove tattoos, tattoos should be considered permanent. Even when they are able to be removed, there may be scarring, and the

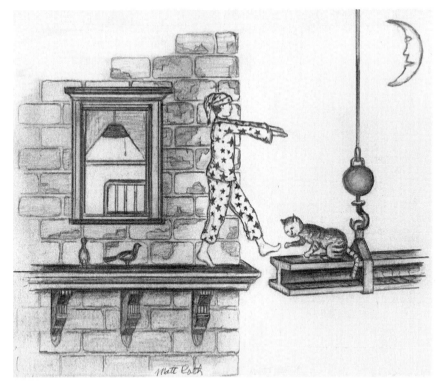

A significant minority of adolescents have at least one episode of sleepwalking. Generally, these episodes are no cause for concern.

procedures are quite expensive and usually not covered by health insurance.

TEMPOROMANDIBULAR JOINT PAIN (TMJ)

The temporomandibular joint is the joint between your jaw and your skull—just in front of your earlobe. When you open and close your jaw, you feel the movement in the joint. Occasionally, teens develop pain in this area, limited jaw movement, or unusual clicks or sounds. If this is a problem, contact your physician or dentist.

TESTICULAR SELF-EXAM (TSE)

Every month, you should check your testicles as follows:

1. During or after a warm shower or bath, use both hands to examine each testicle. Your thumbs should be on top of the testicle, and your index and middle fingers should be on the underside of the testicle.

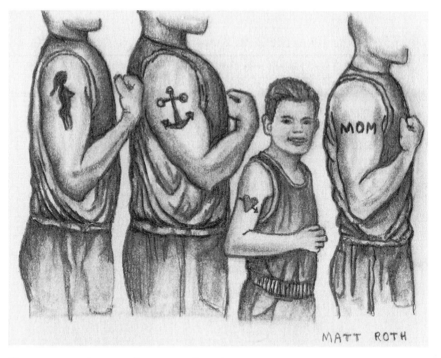

MATT ROTH

You may acquire an infection, such as hepatitis B, by going to an unlicensed tattoo parlor.

2. Roll the testicle between the thumbs and fingers.
3. While you will feel the epididymis as a soft structure at the top and back of each testicle, report any lump, irregularities, or pain to your medical provider.

The purpose of TSE is to detect testicular cancer, which is the most common solid tumor found in young adult males.

TESTICULAR TORSION

This is when the testicle twists around the spermatic cord, leading to persistent moderate or severe pain in the scrotum. In case of testicular torsion, you must see a physician immediately, as emergency surgery is usually needed.

TESTICULAR TUMOR

A testicular tumor is a growth on or in the testicle. Frequently malignant, it requires immediate evaluation. This is why a monthly testicular self-exam is so important.

TESTICLE (UNDESCENDED)

If you have only one testicle in your scrotum, you should notify your physician. You may require treatment to enable the testicle to descend.

URETHRITIS

Urethritis, or the inflammation of the urethra (the tube that connects the bladder to the tip of the penis), is usually caused by a sexually transmitted disease, such as chlamydia or gonorrhea, or a spermicide. Symptoms include pain during urination and a clear, cloudy, yellow, thin, or thick discharge.

VARICOCOELE

A varicocoele is a dilated vein that may be felt above the testicle in the scrotum. It is more frequently found above the left testicle than the right testicle. On standing, a varicocoele may feel like a bag of worms. There may be a sense of fullness in the scrotum or a mild ache. Although surgery is sometimes necessary, most cases do not require any treatment.

ORGANIZATIONS OF INTEREST

American Diabetes Association
1660 Duke Street
Alexandria, VA 22314
800–232–3472

Asthma and Allergy Foundation of America
1125 15th St. NW
Suite 502
Washington, DC 20005
800–727–8462

Crohn's and Colitis Foundation of America
386 Park Avenue South, 17th Floor
New York, NY 10016–8804
800–932–2423

Cystic Fibrosis Foundation
6931 Arlington Road
Bethesda, MD 20814
800–344–4823

National Chronic Fatigue Syndrome Association
3521 Broadway, Suite 222
Kansas City, MO 64111
816–931–4777

National Headache Foundation
428 W. St. James Place, 2nd Floor
Chicago, IL 60614–2750
888-NHF-5552

National Mental Health Association
1021 Prince St.
Alexandria, VA 22314–2971
703–684–7722

National Scoliosis Foundation
5 Cabot Place
Stoughton, MA 02072
800–673–6922

Sickle Cell Disease Association of America
200 Corporate Pointe, Suite 495
Culver City, CA 90230
800–421–8453

WEB SITES OF INTEREST

http://www.drkoop.com This is a Web site with links to many sites dealing with
    health topics.
http://www.adolescenthealth.org This is the Web site for the Society of Adolescent
    Medicine, the professional organization that promotes the development,
    synthesis, and dissemination of knowledge about adolescents.
http://www.aap.org This is the Web site for the American Academy of Pediatrics.
    It has links to sites focusing on many topics of interest to adolescents.
http://www.ama-assn.org This is the Web site for the American Medical Associa-
    tion. It has links to sites related to health topics and fitness.
http://education indiana.edu/cas/adol/adol.htm This is a site for teens, parents, or oth-
    ers interested in adolescents, with excellent links to sites dealing with ad-
    olescent health issues.

HOTLINES AND INFORMATION SOURCES

Hepatitis Helpline
American Liver Foundation

800–223–0179

800–465–4837

HIV/AIDS Hotline

Centers for Disease Control National AIDS Hotline

800–342-AIDS

Impotence Information Center

800–843–4315

Lyme Disease Foundation

800–886–5963

Thyroid Foundation of America, Inc.

800–832–8321

9

Outdoor and Wilderness Health

Early in my career, when I was completing a two-year Public Health Service commitment, I practiced family medicine in the high plateau desert of rural western New Mexico. Between the day and night, there were great fluctuations of temperature. Swings of 60 degrees were not uncommon.

This area of New Mexico had a large percentage of alcoholics. I clearly remember the sad story of a 19-year-old male who had been drinking heavily at one of the many bars in town. Apparently, fairly late in the evening, he had left the bar to walk home—some three miles away. Although it was a frigid January night, he was only dressed in light-weight clothing.

The next morning, he was found partially undressed in a roadside ditch. He had frozen to death. In all probability, the alcohol had made him drowsy and disoriented. Lying down to rest, he had fallen asleep. Within hours, he died from profound hypothermia—an abnormally low body temperature generally caused by a decrease in heat production and excess heat loss.

For optimal functioning, humans, who are warm-blooded animals, need to maintain a relatively stable body temperature. Body heat is produced by the burning of calories for fuel. In healthy adolescent males, a decrease in heat production may be caused by the following:

- Inactivity
- An impairment of the body's thermoregulatory apparatus, such as the ability to shiver

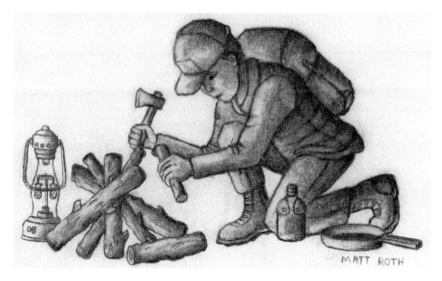

Be certain to keep warm when camping in cold weather.

Excess heat loss may also be caused by environmental factors, including the following:

• Improper dress for the climate
• Wind speed
• Immersion or contact with water
• Lack of adaptation to the climate

It is important to be aware of the symptoms of hypothermia so that you will recognize them in yourself or your friends. Common symptoms include the following:

• Shivering
• Impaired judgment
• Change in mood
• Skin color changes from red to white to blue
• Decreasing level of consciousness

If you notice any of these symptoms, seek a warm shelter and/or medical attention.

Of course, it is best to prevent hypothermia. Always have a partner when you are participating in a risky outside sport, such as cold weather cross-country skiing or hiking. Then you will be able to check on each

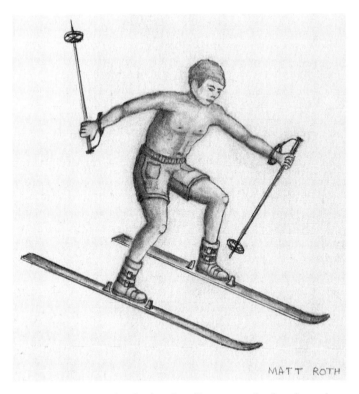

Dressing inappropriately for the climate can lead to hypothermia. Wear effective thermal insulation when engaging in cold-weather activities, and, since significant heat may be lost from your head, be sure to cover it.

other. Wear effective thermal insulation. If your inner garments become wet, change them. Since significant heat may be lost from your head, be sure to cover it. In reference to outdoor clothing, remember the mnemonic COLD.

Clean clothing
Open your clothing to prevent excessive perspiration
Layers of clothing are more effective—they trap warm air
Dry clothing limits the loss of heat

Returning to the adolescent who froze to death, be aware that the alcohol caused him to take risks. It induced sleepiness. And it might have encouraged him to undress. For some unexplained reason, in response to cold, people who have consumed too much alcohol may disrobe. The alcohol also dilated his blood vessels, which caused an increased loss of heat and impaired his ability to shiver. Shivering produces heat. Maybe if his friends had known these facts, this teen would have been alive the next morning.

COLD INJURIES

Frostnip refers to an inconsequential and completely reversible cold-induced injury. The affected body part, usually the fingers or toes, becomes painful. But the pain responds well to simple rewarming procedures.

A more serious condition, *frostbite*, is the freezing of tissue. Frostbite is more likely to occur in those parts of the body directly exposed to cold, such as the earlobes, fingers, toes, and the tip of the nose. Symptoms include numbness, tingling, or a lack of feeling. The skin may become discolored. Since frostbite may destroy tissue and result in complications, it is best treated by a medical provider.

Damage to the cornea of the eyes may occur in high wind-chill situations, such as skiing or snowmobiling. The cornea may actually freeze, leading to eye pain and blurred vision.

Consider the following ways to prevent cold injuries:

• Because heat loss occurs from skin exposed to the elements, dress appropriately. Wear goggles, which may help prevent freezing of the corneas.
• Keep your hands and feet dry.
• Avoid alcohol and tobacco under conditions that could lead to frostbite.
• Mittens are more effective than gloves in maintaining hand warmth.
• Wear clothing which ventilates to prevent excessive perspiration.

Every winter, we hear about people who fall through the ice on a pond. Such an event, known as cold-water immersion, may quickly lead to hypothermia and drowning. Since people who are drinking are more likely to take risks, sometimes alcohol is involved in these dangerous incident. Before taking part in an activity that may lead to cold-water immersion, consider the following questions:

• Do you know how to swim?
• Are you in a good state of health and physical fitness?
• Can you stay levelheaded and not panic in the face of danger?
• Are you wearing protective clothing?
• Is help nearby?
• How warm is the water (warmer is better)?

If there is a chance of cold water immersion, always be with a buddy, do not drink alcohol, and wear appropriate clothing for the weather conditions. All too often, cold-water immersion results in death.

HEAT INJURIES

I recall the case of an 18-year-old ROTC (Reserve Officer Training Corps) candidate who was standing at attention in a formation. It was a bright, sunny, and unusually warm day; the temperature was hovering close to 100 degrees Fahrenheit. Reportedly, he began to sway and then fell to the ground unconscious. His colleagues quickly raised his legs, and, within a minute, he had regained consciousness.

During hot weather, standing erect will increase the amount of blood in your lower extremities, and the heat will cause your blood vessels to dilate, thereby lowering your blood pressure. When your blood pressure falls too low—a figure that varies from person to person—you may lose consciousness. Moving your legs propels the blood to the heart, and may prevent a heat-induced fainting spell.

There are several ways to reduce the chance of heat-induced illness:

- When exercising, wear lightweight and absorbent clothing, such as cotton. Since sweating allows your body to cool, be sure your body surfaces are exposed to the air.
- Acclimate yourself to a hot environment by beginning workouts at a mild to moderate pace and increase the intensity gradually over a ten-day period.
- For every pound lost during exercise, consume an equal amount of fluid.
- Heat-induced injury is based on the outside temperature, humidity, wind speed, and solar radiation as well as the level, type, and duration of exercise. Take all of these factors into consideration when you exercise.

SOLAR HEALTH ISSUES

Solar radiation consists of a number of different wavelengths, including ultraviolet light. Ultraviolet rays cause tanning, burning, premature aging of the skin, and some types of skin cancer. First-degree burns are characterized by redness and pain. If you develop second-degree burns, which are more serious, you'll see disruptions on the skin surface, such as blister formation and peeling, and have a lot of pain. Treatment includes cool compresses, showers, and a variety of over-the-counter preparations. Usually second-degree burns should be treated by a medical provider.

Sunburn can be prevented. Consider the following ways:

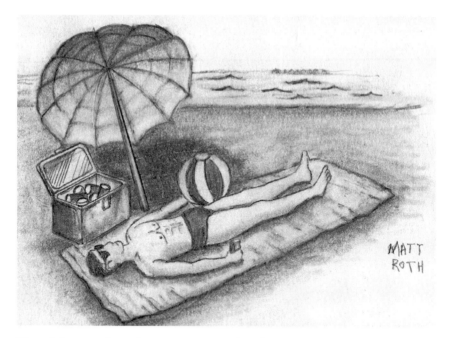

Ultraviolet rays from the sun cause tanning, burning, premature aging of the skin, and some types of skin cancer. You should always put on sunscreen when spending time outdoors.

- Sunburn often occurs early in the summer season before you have a protective tan. The peak hours for UV rays are between 10 A.M. and 2 P.M. Be extra careful during those times.
- Sunscreens contain para-aminobenzoic acid (PABA), which allows you to spend more time in the sun before burning. They are rated with sun protection factor (SPF) numbers. The higher the number, the less likely you will burn. However, an SPF or 15 does not mean you can stay in the sun 15 times longer than someone who does not use sunscreen. Sunburn is not the only consequence of too much sun. Over time, you may experience other skin changes. For example, the risk of skin cancer is correlated with the amount of ultraviolet light you're exposed to. Thus, farmers with light skin who do not use sunscreen have a higher risk of skin cancer than African Americans with desk jobs. Also, years of tanning rays may cause premature aging of the skin.
- Some sunscreens are also waterproof, an obvious advantage if you are swimming or perspiring.
- Teens who burn easily, such as those of Irish or Celtic extraction, or other fair-skinned people, should use sunscreen with an SPF of 30 or higher.
- Most white teens, Asians, and Middle Easterners, who may initially burn but then tan for the remainder of the season, should use sunscreen with a SPF rating of 15.

- African Americans should use an SPF 15–rated sunscreen for outdoor activity.
- Remember, you can also get a severe sunburn in the winter. Be sure to put on sunscreen when you are downhill or cross-country skiing.

Sunblocks use zinc oxide to protect the skin from UV rays. Unfortunately, zinc oxide stains clothing and clogs pores. Clogged pores may lead to pimples. A micronized sunscreen product may be a better choice.

Sunglasses protect your eyes from UV light. This is especially important if you are a skier or mountain climber. People who participate in those sports are susceptible to snowblindness from direct UV rays as well as those reflected off the snow. And the amount of ultraviolet radiation you receive increases the higher the altitude where you're skiing. Under certain conditions, without protection, the corneas of your eyes may burn in less than an hour.

But not all sunglasses are equally effective against UV rays. When selecting sunglasses, review their light transmission and polarization properties. If you participate in water sports, skiing, or mountain climbing, try to find sunglasses that absorb most visible light—up to 95 percent—and *all* ultraviolet light. Polarized lenses decrease the glare from water or snow. Side shields may also be helpful.

WIND ISSUES

Wind may be caused by moving air or by a person moving through the air—such as in cycling. In cold weather, wind is an important source of heat loss.

Thermoregulation, or keeping a normal temperature, may be difficult when it is cold and the wind is blowing rapidly. Wind chill is the term used to describe the rate of cooling. For example, at 30 degrees Fahrenheit, when there is no wind, you will feel cool. However, if there is a wind traveling at five miles per hour, you will feel bitterly cold. Heat is lost by convection, much like cooling off from a fan. The best way to prevent heat loss is to wear multiple layers of clothing made from nylon, cotton nylon, and Gore-Tex. These fabrics trap air and prevent it from moving.

LIGHTNING

Every year, worldwide, there are roughly 1,000 deaths from lighting strikes. Approximately 30 percent of direct lightning hits to humans are fatal. Lightning may cause heart stoppage, seizures, bruises, burns, and confusion. The following precautions may enable you to avoid becoming one of the statistics.

- If you see a thunderstorm approaching, seek shelter in a building or nonconvertible car since these will direct lightning away from your body.
- Stay away from metal objects, appliances, telephones, or computers, which could conduct a lightning bolt.
- If you are out on water, go to the shore immediately and to a structure that will conduct lightning away from you.

PROBLEMS FROM HIGH ALTITUDES

High altitudes may create a number of health problems, such as low oxygen levels in the blood (hypoxia) and acute mountain sickness. Between 5,000 and 10,000 feet of altitude, a teen will experience impairment of exercise performance as well as an increased respiratory effort. From 10,000 to 17,000 feet, the level of oxygen in the blood may be quite low. During sleep and exercise, it may become extremely low. Over 17,000 feet, the oxygen levels may be dangerously low, and, unless an athlete is well acclimated to the environment, supplemental oxygen is usually required.

Thus, in the unlikely event that you were dropped by aircraft on the summit of Mt. Everest, which is 28,000 feet above sea level, you would drift into an unconscious state in only a few minutes. Soon, thereafter, you would die. On the other hand, if you climbed to the summit over a period of days, you would be better acclimated to the lack of oxygen, and you would be at far less risk from oxygen deprivation.

Lack of oxygen affects the nervous system. Typically, people deprived of oxygen experience fatigue, sleepiness, hallucinations, and dizziness. The administration of oxygen may rapidly reverse the symptoms.

Acute mountain illness occurs if you climb up a high altitude—about 7,500 feet or higher—too rapidly. Within eight to 24 hours, you would develop a headache and a loss of appetite, plus dizziness and fatigue. Extreme exertion or consumption of alcohol or tobacco may exacerbate the situation. Heed these ways to prevent acute mountain illness:

- Climb the mountain slowly—no more than 2,000 feet a day.
- Take acetazolamide, a diuretic, before beginning the ascent. This medication rapidly enhances ventilatory acclimatization and also helps to maintain oxygenation during sleep.
- Avoid alcohol for at least 24 hours before climbing and the first two nights at high altitude.
- Eat a diet that is at least 70 percent carbohydrates.

HEALTH PROBLEMS FROM HIGH WATER PRESSURE

For every 32 feet of water depth you descend, the pressure on your body increases one atmosphere. Therefore, if you are a scuba diver and

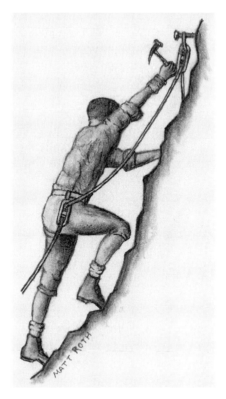

Mountain climbing is an activity attractive to teens, but there can be problems due to altitude sickness.

you dive 50 feet, you are surrounded by pressure that is 1.5 times stronger than normal. This increase in water pressure may cause medical problems such as barotrauma, in which the eardrum is pushed inward. If you have a cold, you may not be able to equalize the pressure, and this could result in a ruptured eardrum. Injury from water pressure may also affect your inner ear and your sinuses. Ask your scuba instructor how to prevent these problems.

BURN INJURIES

I remember the first patient I saw when I practiced medicine in rural upstate New York. While riding his motorcycle, this 18-year-old accidentally placed his bare lower leg on the exhaust pipe. The significant burn that he sustained was about an inch in diameter, the flesh was black, and he lost feeling in the area. This was a third-degree burn. Treat-

ment included careful cleaning of the wound, topical application of antibiotic ointments, and frequent observation for a month. If he had worn
protective clothing, he could have prevented this injury.

During camping or other outdoor activities, you may be susceptible
to burn injuries. First-degree burns usually result in redness and pain;
no blisters are formed. Second-degree burns are accompanied by blisters
and fluid collection, and there is pain. Third-degree burns are deeper,
and healing and treatment are more complicated. The pain from a burn
injury is often relieved by immersing the burned area in cold water.

When discussing burns, remember the following points:

- If you or one of your friends is on fire, *do not run!!* Instead, force the victim to
lie down and keep the flames away from his face. Douse him with cold water.
Take off the burned clothing to prevent further injury *Seek medical attention
immediately.*

- For an electrical burn, be absolutely certain not to touch the victim until the
electrical current is turned off. Basic cardiopulmonary resuscitation may be
necessary. *Seek medical attention immediately.*

- Chemical burns need to be flushed with copious amounts of water. Flush for
at least five to ten minutes. *Seek medical attention immediately.*

- Scald burns are caused by hot water or other liquids. At 156 degrees Fahrenheit,
you may receive a significant second-degree burn after one second of contact
with hot liquid. Be sure to remove any clothing that has absorbed the hot liquid,
and flush the burns with lots of cold water. Based on the size of the burn, you
may need to seek medical attention.

HEALTH ISSUES INVOLVING WATER AND WATER SPORTS

There are a number of injuries and illnesses associated with outdoor
water activities. In salt water, injuries may occur both from the environment and from saltwater animals. The first time I snorkeled in a beautiful
sun-drenched cove in the British Virgin Islands, I scraped my hand
against a coral reef. I felt immediate pain, which was followed by swelling. Fortunately, with proper cleaning, none of the scrapes became infected.

Sharks have a very sensitive sense of smell and may detect minute
amounts of blood or urine in the water. Further, they hear prey from a
distance of 3,000 feet. Tiger sharks, great white sharks, and hammerhead
sharks may attack humans. To avoid a shark attack, take the following
precautions:

- Do not swim in shark-infested waters.
- Since sharks tend to attack solitary swimmers, swim in groups.

- If you are bleeding, do not go into any area where there may be sharks. And do not spear a fish. Sharks are attracted to fish blood too.
- Sharks are drawn to bright-colored bathing suits (such as orange). Black suits are reported to be the least attractive.
- Avoid swimming with shiny, dangling jewelry. Sharks will swim toward it.

Many varieties of jellyfish sting. The stings may produce redness, pain, and swelling. The box jellyfish, which is found in waters off Queensland, Australia, is an extremely deadly type of jellyfish. After being stung, humans have been known to die within 30 seconds.

The Portuguese man-of-war is an organism up to 12 inches long with tentacles that have been measured up to 100 feet. The man-of-war seems to abound in tropical waters of the Atlantic Ocean especially off of the coasts of Florida and Mexico. The tentacles are transparent, and if they happen to touch you, they will discharge their contents into you. The victim can get red and painful stings.

Despite its name, the stingray, a fish found in warm and shallow ocean waters, stings only defensively, so it will not bother you unless you bother it. Thus, if you happen to step on a stingray, it may thrust its tail (stinger) into your foot. Venom will be released. It has been reported that the tail of a stingray is able to pierce leather, rubber, or even wood. Be careful when you are walking in shallow waters that may be inhabited by stingrays.

You may also be harmed by leeches—especially in fresh water. Leeches bite and inject an anticoagulant. Bleeding occurs quickly and without pain. The engorged leech may then fall off. If you notice a leech biting you, pour a few drops of alcohol, vinegar, or salt water near the point of attachment. That encourages it to fall off. Do not pull it off. The jaws could remain imbedded in your skin and would require minor surgery to remove them.

A few skin infections are caused by exposure to water. If your canal is moist for long periods of time, you may develop swimmer's ear, an infection of the ear canal between the earlobe and the eardrum. In cases of swimmer's ear, bacteria create an infection, accompanied by pain, swelling, and discharge. Prescription ear drops are helpful. But, as always, it is better to prevent swimmer's ear. Keep your ear canals as dry as possible. (But never put cotton swabs in the canals.) Tilting you head to one side and shaking the water out removes water.

People who use hot tubs or outdoor whirlpools are susceptible to a condition called hot tub dermatitis, a skin infection caused by the bacterium pseudomonas. Due to improper disinfection methods, some hot tubs have high concentrations of this bacteria. This bacteria may attack normal skin and cause a bumpy, red, itchy rash. It you think you have this problem, consult your healthcare provider. Treatment for this infection usually requires oral antibiotics.

Certain hazards are associated with whitewater sports. The most common injuries stemming from whitesports are fractures, shoulder dislocations, near drownings, leg injuries, and lacerations. If you suffer an injury that breaks the surface of the skin, you run the risk of infection. A protozoan known as Giardia lamblia, which is frequently found in freshwater streams, is excreted in the feces of animals (including humans) and causes a moderately severe diarrhea disease in humans. Also, during whitewater activities, you may easily swallow water. Since Giardia is tasteless and odorless, it is easy to be infected through oral ingestion. If you have protracted or severe diarrhea, be sure to contact your medical provider.

People who participate in whitewater sports are also at risk for sunburn and hypothermia from cold-water immersion. And exposure to poison-ivy vines and other plants along the shore may cause contact dermatitis. Typically, the poison-ivy rash is red, irregular, and bubbly in appearance. It is best treated with anti-itch medications, and, if necessary, steroid creams or pills. Familiarize yourself with the appearance of the poison ivy plant. If you are exposed, wash the area thoroughly with soap and water.

STINGS AND BITES

I recall the case of a 14-year-old patient who had an encounter with a yellow-faced hornet. Within 20 minutes, he broke out in itchy hives and began having difficulty breathing. Soon, he collapsed and was rushed to the nearest hospital. There he received adrenalin, steroids, and intravenous fluids. Thankfully, he recovered. After consulting with an allergist, he was given monthly antiwasp treatments. He was also instructed to always carry an injection of adrenalin, which he could self-administer if he were ever stung again. Thus far, he has remained healthy.

There are a wide variety of stinging or biting insects. Many are simply a nuisance; others are potentially dangerous. Let's review some of the more common ones.

Bees, Fire Ants, and Wasps

These insects are members of the order Hymenoptera. Most are social insects; so disturbing a nest may bring on a community attack. Generally, they sting on provocation. It is well known that fruit or fruit syrup attracts yellow jackets; painting or working along the outside of a house may incite a wasp attack; and rain may draw fire ants to your home.

The venom injected from the stinger of one of these insects has toxins, enzymes, and other substances that destroy cells, trigger a histamine response from the body, and cause intense pain. Histamine is a chemical produced by your body that causes your skin to swell, itch, and turn red. Most people have localized reactions to the stings. However, as in the case of my patient, there may be systemic reactions as well. Because these stings may be life threatening, they must always be evaluated by your medical provider. Fatalities—thankfully rare—have been reported from African killer bee attacks. These aggressive insects are only found in South and Central America as well as sections of Texas, Arizona, and southern California.

Here are some strategies to prevent stings:

- Be aware of where the nests are located and avoid those areas.
- Wear protective gear, such as gloves or a hood over your face, when working around these areas.
- Avoid wearing bright-colored clothing, colognes, and fruity scents. These may all attract the insects.
- Walking barefoot in areas where these insects live is asking for trouble.

Mosquitoes, Blackflies, Fleas, Ticks, and Chiggers

All these insects bite to suck blood, which is their food. You are most at risk for a mosquito bite at dawn and dusk during the warmer months of the year. Body heat, carbon dioxide, and lactic acid, which is a by-product of exercise, are known to entice mosquitoes. Their bite is relatively benign. Often, you feel the bite as the mosquito is biting. That is followed by several hours of an itchy sensation. These hints may help you avoid mosquito bites.

- Do not go into infested areas at dawn and/or dusk.
- Wear a repellent such as DEET or insecticide such as permethrins. DEET discourages the insect from landing on you. Permethrins kill the landed insect. Read the label carefully and follow the directions to the letter.
- Cover as much of your skin as possible with clothing.

Blackflies bite only during the day. Although you do not feel the bite, the itch is more intense and longer lasting than that caused by mosquitoes. Blackflies are even known to crawl under clothing to bite. Follow the protective points noted above for mosquitoes.

Fleas suck blood from warm-blooded animals such as dogs, cats, and humans. The flea bite is itchier and longer lasting than the mosquito bite. While DEET repels fleas, you should contact your veterinarian if your pet or room is infested.

Not only do ticks bite, but they also transmit microorganisms that cause disease. Two of the most common diseases spread by tick bites are Lyme disease and Rocky Mountain Spotted Fever. Lyme disease is spread by the deer tick, which is about the size of a pin head. Dog ticks and wood ticks spread Rocky Mountain Spotted Fever. Unfed, these are the size of a match head. When filled with blood, they may swell to the size of a jelly bean. If you are bitten by a tick and are not sure of the species, save it for further evaluation. Try these safeguards to prevent tick bites.

- In areas known to have ticks, wear clothing tucked in at your shoes.
- Use an insect repellent, such as DEET.
- When in an infested area, have a body inspection twice daily.
- Know the appearance of the ticks that populate your area of the country.
- Learn how to properly and safely remove biting ticks. Never squeeze or crush ticks when you remove them. The best method is to use tweezers. Apply the tweezers to the tick's body as close to the skin and mouthparts as possible. Gently pull straight back opposite to the direction that the mouthparts are entering into the skin. With slow and gentle traction, the entire tick and mouthparts should come out. Clean the wound with soap and water. If you do not have tweezers and must use your fingers, then wear gloves or protect your fingers with facial tissue. Wash your hands after removal of the tick.

For people 15 and older, there is a vaccine to help prevent Lyme disease. Contact your physician for more information on this series of three injections.

Chiggers are blood-sucking insects that bite humans—commonly on the legs or feet—during part of the insect's life cycle. Chigger larvae live on vegetation waiting for a host to walk by. Once they attach to a host, they bite and feed on blood. The bite is very itchy and red. Symptoms may last for weeks. If symptoms become severe, they should be evaluated by a medical provider. DEET or permethrins, sprayed on clothing, may repel chigger larvae.

Spider bites, especially those from the brown recluse or black widow spiders, may be life threatening. Brown spiders are light to dark brown in color and have a violin-shaped spot that begins on their heads and travels down their backs. These spiders inhabit woodpiles and emerge at night during the warmer months to capture insects. Their bite has a venom that may cause red blood cells to burst. Frequently victims of brown spider bites experience a localized skin reaction. But serious symptoms—such as fever, headache, vomiting, and blood or kidney problems—may also occur. The black widow is identified by a red hourglass on her abdomen, a sharp contrast to her black body color. Found in barns, outbuildings, and trash piles, the black widow will bite if her web is disturbed. A black widow's bite is intensely painful and may send muscles into spasm within 30 to 60 minutes. Medical assistance should be sought immediately.

Though scorpions thrive in many warm areas of the country, they are most common in the Southwest. The bite of a southwestern desert scorpion may cause localized pain and swelling and impair the functioning of nerves and muscles. In more serious cases, a bite may result in blurred vision, slurred speech, shaking, and jerking. Medical assistance should be obtained immediately. Spraying an area with insecticides has been known to kill scorpions. In scorpion-infested areas, be sure to shake your clothes and shoes before putting them on.

Centipedes have fangs that inject venom. After a bite, you will experience pain, redness, and swelling that may persist for several weeks. These bites are treated with medications that address their symptoms, including calamine lotion. Millipedes have two pairs of legs per body segment. They do not bite. Instead, they secrete fluids that burn and blister human skin. Do not handle millipedes without protective clothing.

Bites from Reptiles and Mammals

Reptiles

According to the American Association of Poison Control Systems, in 1992 there were 4,675 reports of poisonous and nonpoisonous snake bites in the United States. One person died from such a bite. Most snake bites occur during the warmer months. Of all sectors of the population, young adult males are most likely to be bitten.

Pit vipers, which include cottonmouths, copperheads, and rattlesnakes, are the most prevalent poisonous snakes in the United States and account for 95 percent of snake bites. The poisonous venom of one of these vipers may destroy muscle, red blood cells, and other tissues. Signs of a poisonous bite include pain, redness, swelling, vomiting, weakness, low blood pressure, and tissue death. All poisonous or possibly poisonous snake bites must be evaluated by medical personnel. There are several key ways to avoid poisonous snake bites:

• Since most snakes bite people on the hands and feet, wear protective clothing, especially leather boots and gloves.

• Avoid areas where snakes live, including rocky ledges, wood or rock piles, caves, and deserted buildings.

• Do not reach into dark areas where you can't see anything.

There are two poisonous lizards in the United States—the Gila monster and the Mexican beaded lizard. They are both found in southern Arizona. Follow the precautions noted above to avoid snake bites. The Gila monster may doggedly hang on to its victim, and crowbars or pliers may be needed to remove it.

Mammals

As we were preparing to leave our cabin in rural Maine for our home outside Boston, I tried to place Clementine, our family cat, in her traveling crate. Clementine, who had always been quite docile, had other plans. She bit into the flesh between my left thumb and index finger and tenaciously held onto my hand. It took some effort to loosen her jaw. Even though I thoroughly washed the bite, within two hours it began to throb. Mouth bacteria from Clementine had apparently been injected into my hand. This bacteria, Pasteurella multocida, may trigger a virulent infection. It took a solid week of double antibiotics before I saw improvement. My lesson: Wear leather gloves when handling a potentially upset domestic animal.

There are a number of other mammalian bites that you can sustain from outdoor activities. Dogs, rats, skunks, bats, and even humans are some of the animals that inflict bite wounds on humans. Considering the seriousness of rabies, dog bites may be life threatening. A physician or veterinarian may help evaluate the risks by assessing whether the dog is domesticated or wild, whether the bite was a response to provocation, and the dog's history of rabies vaccinations.

Rats are more often found in urban locations. Although they tend to shy away from humans, they do forage at night for food, and they will bite if they feel threatened. Rat bites transmit an organism that causes rat-bite fever, a disease characterized by fever, chills, rash, and arthritis.

Obviously, skunk bites are rare. Since each skunk has a sac around its anus that secretes a noxious odor, you will almost certainly be sprayed long before you are sufficiently close to be bitten. Should you be sprayed, use tomato juice on your clothing and skin to remove the odor. If you are bitten by a skunk, seek immediate medical attention. The skunk could be rabid.

Bat bites may also be dangerous. Vampire bats, which sleep during the day but are active at night, suck blood to live. A vampire bat requires one ounce of blood per day as food. This blood may be from a human or another mammal. If you are camping, use mosquito netting to protect yourself. Bats do carry rabies, so any bat bite should be looked at by a physician.

Human bites carry bacteria and may transmit other diseases, including herpes, hepatitis, and tuberculosis. Since infection may readily occur, human bites to the hand are potentially quite harmful. They need medical evaluation with possible antibiotic treatment.

DANGERS FROM PLANTS

Teens who are active outdoors may incur disease from plants, including skin rashes, irritation, and poisoning. Poison ivy and poison oak are the most common plants causing skin rashes.

I vividly recall the teen who came to see me because of a rash around his anus. He had been camping in the forest without any sanitary facilities or supplies. Since he failed to bring along toilet tissue, he used the leaves of a shiny vine to wipe himself. Within hours, he had a red, burning, itchy poison ivy rash around his anus. To say the least, he was not a happy camper.

Poison ivy and poison oak are found in the lower 48 states. Generally, there are three leaves attached to the same point in the stem. Most people are not violently sensitive to these plants. If you wash the skin well within two to four hours of exposure, you may prevent a reaction. Severe reactions should be seen by a physician, who may prescribe topical or oral steroids.

There are many blackberry plants around our house and in the nearby conservation land. I have sustained innumerable wounds from blackberry thorns. The best treatment is thorough washing of the area punctured by the thorn. Long-sleeved shirts and long trousers help prevent these injuries. Some plants have hairs that may cause hives in victims. And some people are very sensitive to contact with certain plants, such as chives, onions, or even lettuce. They may have an allergic reaction from direct exposure.

Socrates died from hemlock poisoning. Ingestion of certain plants, such as jimsonweed, may result in anticholinergic syndrome. These plants contain chemical compounds which interfere with your ability to perspire and salivate. They also induce your pupils and blood vessels to dilate and cause some individuals to become mentally disoriented. Medical students memorize the symptoms of the anticholinergic syndrome:

(The patient is)

- Hot as a hare
- Blind as a bat
- Dry as a bone
- Red as a beet
- Mad as a hatter

Victims of this type of poisoning lose their ability to sweat, their pupils dilate, they become dehydrated and flushed, and they experience changes in their behavior. Hence, the medical student mnemonic above.

While there are over 40,000 species of mushrooms, only a small number are poisonous. The problem is that the average person may not be able to identify the deadly ones. This should be left to the experts. Poisonous mushrooms may cause problems with your digestive system, vomiting, behavioral changes, seizures, or even liver or kidney failure. Always seek immediate medical attention if you develop any symptoms after eating wild mushrooms. But, unless you have consulted an expert, it is best not to eat them in the first place.

INFECTIONS FROM THE OUTDOORS

A number of infections may be acquired during outdoor activities. These include traveler's diarrhea, malaria, yellow fever, hepatitis A, cholera, typhoid fever, salmonella, and shigella. These will be reviewed in the next chapter, on life issues.

REFERENCES

Auerbach, Paul S., editor. *Wilderness Medicine: Management of Wilderness and Environmental Emergencies*. 3rd edition. St. Louis: Mosby, 1995.

Fields, Karl B., and Peter Fricker, editors. *Medical Problems in Athletes*. Oxford, England: Blackwell Science, 1997.

Herman, Bruce E., and Elisabeth G. Skokan. "Bites That Poison. A Tale of Spiders, Snakes, and Scorpions." *Contemporary Pediatrics* 16 (August 1999) 8: 41–62.

Madda, Frank C., editor. *Outdoor Emergency Medicine*. Chicago: Contemporary Books, Inc. 1982.

McAnarney, Elizabeth, Richard Kreipe, Donald Orr, and George Comerci, editors. *Textbook of Adolescent Medicine*. Philadelphia: W. B. Saunders Co., 1992.

10

Life Issues

TRAVEL

Thanks to drastically discounted student airfares, increasing numbers of U.S. teens are traveling to other countries. While interacting with people from other cultures and societies is clearly quite valuable in terms of personal growth, you must realize that foreign travel may expose you to a host of new illnesses. Before you begin your journey, you need to take the time to determine if you will require immunizations in advance or you will need to take along special medications.

The most common illness acquired while traveling is "traveler's diarrhea," which is caused by the Escherichia coli bacteria. You contract traveler's diarrhea by ingesting food or water contaminated with fecal matter. Typically, the illness begins during the first week of travel and occurs more often in younger travelers, such as teens. Symptoms include watery stools, bloating, nausea, cramps, fever, and fatigue. The most risky destinations for traveler's diarrhea are the developing countries, including those in Latin America, and southern Europe. If someone tells you not to drink the local water, don't. Drink only bottled water or other bottled beverages, hot tea, or hot coffee. Also remember to brush your teeth and wash all fruits and vegetables with bottled water before eating them.

Nevertheless, if you do become ill, Imodium or Pepto-Bismol may bring some relief from the symptoms. Your physician can also prescribe an antibiotic, such as ciprofloxacin or Bactrim, to treat the diarrhea.

While you may be exposed to bites and stings from a variety of animals in other countries, it is particularly important to stay away from

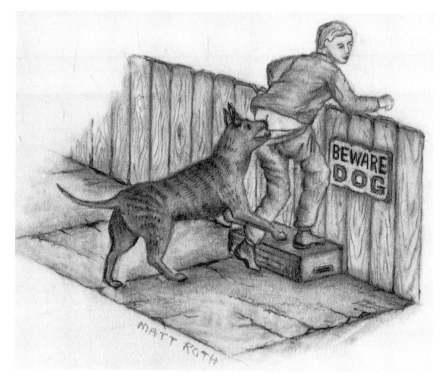

Dog bites may transmit diseases, so it's important to be seen by a medical professional immediately after being bitten.

wild animals, including monkeys. In certain countries, rabies may be endemic. So, in these high-risk areas, avoid dogs, cats, or other animals. If you sustain an animal bite, seek medical attention. Unless you plan to be in a rural area of a country where rabies is endemic, rabies vaccinations are generally not necessary.

I have given sterile disposable syringes and needles to some teens who plan to travel in rural parts of developing nations especially in areas where there is an increased prevalence of HIV (the sub-Sahara region in Africa, for instance). Then, if those teens need an injection, they can ask the local medical provider to use the safe syringe and needle. Also be sure to bring along a prescription for the syringes and needles. You do not want authorities to think that you are carrying them for any illegal purposes.

Swimming in contaminated or dirty water may be dangerous. In some countries, bodies of water may contain human or dog feces, and you can easily contract a viral or bacterial infection or hepatitis A from swimming in such contaminated water. In addition, parasites abound in such settings. If you have any concerns about the safety of a body of water, don't swim in it. Only chlorinated water is considered a relatively safe place to swim.

You need to discuss vaccinations with your medical provider. Even if you do not travel, adolescent males should be up-to-date for hepatitis B, tetanus-diphtheria, polio, measles, mumps, and rubella immunizations. In order for teens to travel in Canada and most Western European countries, they need have only those vaccinations that are required to attend U.S. schools.

But travel to other countries may be far riskier and requires additional vaccinations and medications. Some of the vaccines that you may be required to have are the following:

Hepatitis A

The hepatitis A vaccine prevents this infectious disease of the liver, which is acquired by ingesting food or water contaminated with human feces. For teens, the vaccine is given in two doses; the second dose is administered 6 to 12 months following the first dose. About 2 to 4 weeks after the first dose, the body begins to acquire some protection against the disease.

Typhoid

The typhoid vaccine protects against an infection from the bacteria Salmonella typhi, which causes typhoid fever. Typhoid fever is spread by contaminated food or water. Most experts recommend giving the vaccine to people traveling to Latin America, Africa, and Asia. I prescribe the oral form of the vaccine, which is given as a pill every other day for a total of four doses at least two weeks prior to departure. The vaccine protects against typhoid fever for about five years.

Yellow Fever

Typically, yellow fever, which is transmitted by mosquitoes, is seen in tropical South America and in an area around the equator in Africa. Effective for 10 years, the vaccine must be given at least 10 days prior to your arrival in an infected area.

Meningococcal disease

Certain areas of Africa regularly experience epidemics of meningococcal disease, a bacterial disease that is transmitted when people live in close quarters. Your medical provider should check the current infor-

mation on the incidence of meningococcal disease in the region where
you plan to travel. A single dose of vaccine is available; immunity lasts
about five years.

Cholera

Cholera is a terrible disease in which the patient suffers from severe
dehydrating diarrhea. It can be fatal. Unfortunately, there is no effective
preventative vaccine. Avoid drinking water contaminated with human
feces. Cholera outbreaks have been reported in Latin America, Africa,
and Asia.

Malaria

Malaria, which has been reported in many countries in Africa, Latin
America, Asia, and the Pacific Rim, is caused by protozoa spread
through the bite of a mosquito. If you are traveling to a country where
malaria is prevalent, you should take along prophylactic medications.
Although chloroquine has frequently been prescribed, the malaria organism is now showing a resistance to it. As a result, mefloquine is now
generally prescribed for travelers to chloroquine-resistant malaria areas.
This medication is taken once a week. Begin taking the pill before you
start your travels. Continue taking it weekly while you are there and for
four weeks after you return.

Physicians generally suggest that patients travel with medications that
they may potentially need. You should have medicines for diarrhea and
cramps as well as respiratory illnesses and headaches. Taking along a
balanced electrolyte mix of salts and water or solution for diarrhea is
also a good idea. If you become sick in a foreign country, do not hesitate
to seek medical help. The U.S. State Department has lists of qualified
physicians in every country. Or you can always contact the closest U.S.
embassy.

For further information on vaccinations for foreign travel, consult the
Centers for Disease Control Web site: *www.cdc.gov*. There you will be
able to check the vaccinations required for all the countries on your itin-
erary.

Other travel-related issues may arise while you are out of the country.
Everyone knows that pickpockets are ubiquitous and that certain crim-
inals target tourists. That is why it is always better to travel with at least
one other person. And, of course, use common sense. For example, because of an active volcano producing lava flows, there is an alert in the
Mexican states of Jalisco and Colima. And the Middle East countries
have historically been the site for terrorist actions.

Do not even consider possessing, using, or selling illicit drugs. In some countries, punishments for such actions may be quite severe, and living conditions in the prisons may be close to unbearable. It is not uncommon for both male and female prostitutes to have a high prevalence of HIV. Do not have sex with them. Such actions may have serious—even deadly—consequences. To access safety information from the U.S. State Department, check the following Web site: *http//travel.state.gov/ travel_warnings html.*

ALTERNATIVE OR COMPLEMENTARY MEDICINE

It seems that just about every day the news media report some new piece of information about alternative or complementary medicine. What are those areas of healthcare, and do they have any relevance to you as an adolescent male?

One way to understand the concept of alternative or complementary medicine is to review the treatments for asthma, a common respiratory ailment in male adolescents. Asthma is a chronic inflammation of the bronchi, the air-carrying tubes between your lungs and windpipe, which may develop as a result of allergy or other stimuli. This causes a "hyper response" from the respiratory system. When that happens, your bronchi constrict (known as bronchoconstriction), and your airflow becomes obstructed. You then experience asthma symptoms, such as difficulty in breathing, wheezing, and shortness of breath.

Traditionally, practitioners of Western medicine treat asthma by prescribing medications that reduce bronchial inflammation, prevent bronchoconstriction, and bring on bronchodilation (opening of the bronchi). Many well-controlled studies have supported the effectiveness of this approach. An inhaled steroid medication, such as triamcinolone, reduces inflammation. Albuterol, another inhaled medication, which has stimulatory effects, reverses bronchoconstriction. Cromolyn and nedocromil, other inhaled medications, decrease the hyperresponsiveness of the bronchi. A relatively new class of oral medications, called leukotriene modifiers, may reduce swelling and mucus in the bronchi. All these medications have toxicities or side effects, but these can be monitored by your physician, and the medication dose or type may be adjusted as needed.

There are alternative or complementary treatments for asthma as well. Let's begin with herbal remedies, which, incidentally, are not regulated by the U.S. Food and Drug Administration. In Europe, gingko biloba is widely used to control asthma. A small pilot study, published in 1987, found that gingko biloba was protective against exercise-induced asthma. However, there are no long-term studies of its effectiveness. In addition, vitamin B6 seems to improve some asthma patient's ability to exhale (Collipp, Goldzier, Weiss, et al., 1975).

Alternative or complementary medicine also advocates changes in life-style. For example, practitioners will advise their patients with asthma to exercise. A noncontrolled review of asthmatic children who had weekly swimming practice throughout the winter found improvements in the amount of the air they exhaled over a short period of time, termed the *peak flow*. Meanwhile, a controlled study of yoga training in young adults found that those who practiced yoga developed greater tolerance for exercise and required fewer medications (Vedanthan et al., 1998).

And how about an alternative therapy such as massage? Children with asthma whose parents massaged them for 20 minutes before bedtime reportedly had improved lung functioning. Perhaps massage reduces stress or the anxiety triggers of asthma (Field et al., 1998).

Therapies—such as acupuncture, healing touch, prayer, and home-opathy—also have their share of adherents. No studies on adolescents prove that either prayer or homeopathy reduce the symptom of asthma. One study of acupuncture found that it was helpful in preventing exercise-induced asthma (Fung et al., 1986). But another study found no benefit. In a small German study, in which 12 patients received healing touch over an eight-week period, there appeared to be some improve-ment, and a few of the subjects required less medication (Wacker, 1996).

As a consumer, you must realize that many alternative therapies for asthma have not been proven effective. That does not mean they are not effective—just that there is no clear proof of their effectiveness. You should consult your medical provider. Some of the therapies—such as swimming, yoga, and massage—may easily complement Western treat-ments. Using them may enable patients to use less medication.

There are many alternative medicine therapies that are utilized to re-duce stress. A brief review of several of these methods is useful since stress is a source of concern for many adolescent males.

Acupressure. Acupressure is a technique where light to medium pressure, usu-ally from fingers or hands, is applied to acupoints. Reportedly, stimulation of these points helps to relax muscles, allows blood to flow more freely, and frees an emotional block by releasing accumulated tension.

Acupuncture. Although acupuncture has been part of medical practice in China for about 4,500 years, it is relatively new to the United States. Inserting needles and applying heat or electrical stimulation at very precise acupuncture points, according to advocates of acupuncture, may relieve certain symptoms such as muscle tension and stress.

Aromatherapy. In aromatherapy, concentrated extracts from plants are inhaled or massaged into the body. An emotional response to the aroma can create a relaxed and comfortable response from the body.

Bodywork. In bodywork, techniques are utilized which promote relaxation es-pecially of the musculoskeletal system. These techniques include lessons in

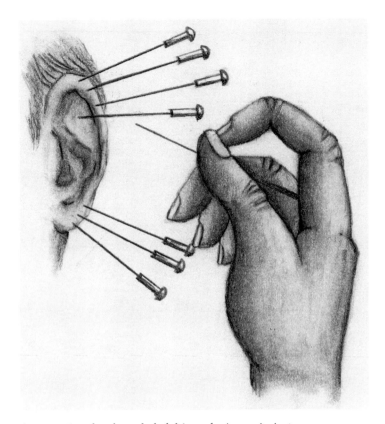

Acupuncture has been helpful in reducing pain in teens.

proper movement and posture, exercise, massage, and other forms of body manipulation.

Flower remedies. Edward Bach developed flower remedies in the late 1920s and 1930s. Using extracts of certain flowers, which are placed under the tongue, Bach taught that this may be useful for a variety of situations, including stress relief, negative moods, and loneliness.

Herbal medicine. Herbal medicine probably dates back to China for at least 2,500 years. Many teens are familiar with St. John's Wort, which has been promoted for depression. In fact, this herbal medication contains chemicals that act in the same way as some antidepressants.

Light Therapy. Light therapy is proven to be effective for Seasonal Affective Disorder (SAD). Like many other medical problems, SAD is aggravated by stress. Appropriate treatment of SAD with light therapy will diminish stress.

Massage. Massage has been an effective therapy for muscle injuries for thousands of years. But it also has important emotional and psychological benefits as it relaxes muscles and in turn reduces stress.

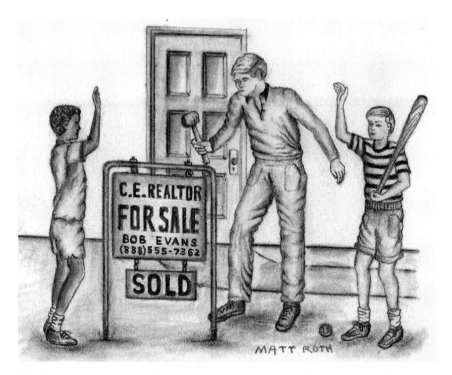

Moving to a new town often causes teens stress, as they terminate close relationships in one town and have to make new friends in another.

Meditation. Meditation is a practice described as resting while remaining awake
    and alert. Teens may meditate while they sit quietly with closed eyes. It is
    recommended for stress and painful conditions.
Reflexology. Reflexology is a discipline in which it is believed there are zones
    and reflex areas in the feet and hands, which correspond to glands, organs,
    and systems of the body. Applying pressure using thumb, finger, or hand
    techniques to these reflex areas will result in the reduction of stress.

STRESS

These are stressful times for teens. This is due, in part, to the fast pace
of our modern society, the complexities of a highly technological society,
and the breakup of the traditional family unit. In addition, today's
youths have more freedom in areas such as time management, sexual
expression, and access to money.

You may experience stress from your family, school, peers, job, community, society, or because of some global event. Stressors commonly
reported by teens include arguments in the family, serious family illness,
breakup with girlfriends or boyfriends, failing grades, personal illness,

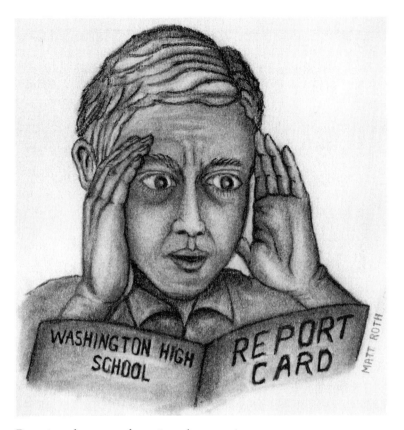

Report cards can produce stress in many teens.

moving, changing schools, and death of a parent (or other close relative) or a close friend.

When faced with stress, we must respond and adapt. That requires physical and emotional energy. But stress is not always a negative force. Training for a marathon may be stressful, for instance, but it should also be a positive experience.

To cope with stress, remember how muscle training works. To build muscles through exercise, you have to stress your muscles. Then you go through a period of relaxation and recovery. To create more strength, you repeat this cycle. You should take the same approach to the stressors in your life. Throughout your life, you will face stresses. To deal with them, you will need to take time for relaxation and recovery. Some teens, who grapple with chronic stress, experience physical symptoms ranging from fatigue and headaches to gastrointestinal problems. For them, it might be wise to consult a counseling professional or take a course in stress reduction or yoga.

You will deal with stress better if you learn time-management skills. This means keeping an orderly schedule of your various life activities. And this schedule should include time to vent your emotions. While males are less likely than females to talk to their friends and families about their feelings, I would encourage such discussions. Confide in someone you trust—a close friend, teacher, or family member. Many male teens also relieve stress through physical activities, such as a sport or another outside interest. Karate and meditation are also useful stress relievers. On the other hand, it is maladaptive to use substances such as alcohol to reduce stress levels.

No one leads a stress-free life. Stress is unavoidable. That is why you need to develop skills to cope with stress. Keep in mind that these coping strategies will undoubtedly change as you pass through the different stages of life.

VIOLENCE

Littleton, Colorado. April 20, 1999. Much has been written about the causes of this horrendous tragedy perpetrated by male teens. Access to guns, youth culture, poor adaptation skills, and many other factors blended together to trigger this tragic sequence of events. What is clear is that for Eric Harris and Dylan Klebold, the two perpetrators, fantasies of rage and violence became real in part because they found in each other kindred spirits. Isolated and alienated from the majority of their peers, these teens had intense rage brewing inside them, and they experienced an erosion of their conscience and means of self-control. While many teens may have violent emotions and fantasies, the vast majority learn to sort through and deal with their feelings. This may not be an easy task. Teens are bombarded with images of violence from movies and television, creating the illusion that violence is the norm. It is not.

During your teen years, you will be exposed to violence in television programming, films, the newspaper, and everyday events that could happen to you. Research studies have shown that the most significant factor leading to violent behavior is youthful exposure to violence. And, repeatedly, studies have demonstrated that there is a link between exposure to media violence and subsequent violent behavior. As children and adolescents witness violent behavior through the various forms of media, they are taught to act aggressively toward others. Moreover, as the exposure continues, they become desensitized to violence and are more fearful of being victimized. As a result, some children and adolescents respond aggressively to conflicts and are more accepting of violence and less caring toward others.

According to an article by Michael Rich, M.D., an adolescent specialist at the Division of Adolescent Medicine at Children's Hospital in Boston,

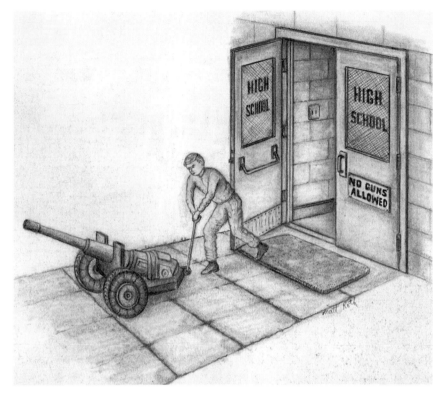

A sense of isolation and alienation and feelings of rage may prompt male teens to turn to violence.

about 75 percent of 12–19-year-old adolescents spend an average of six hours a week watching music videos. Music videos, and other forms of mass media, have in turn become "superpeers," which are all too often taking the place traditionally assumed by friends and family. Instead of modeling their behavior after friends and family, adolescents are modeling it after people in the media.

That is why Renee Hobbs of Babson College in Wellesley, Massachusetts, believes that it is important for young people to become "media literate." Such literacy entails an ability to do the following:

- Determine who is the author and what is the purpose of a media message.
- Determine the techniques that are used to attract viewers' attention.
- Determine the lifestyle and points of view that are represented.
- Determine how different people might interpret the message.
- Determine what has been omitted from the message.

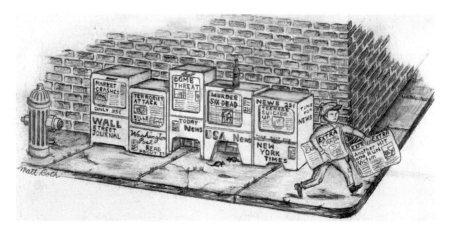

Research studies have shown that the most significant determinant of violent behavior is youthful exposure to violence.

One of my patients was bullied by several other eighth graders for no apparent reason. After coaching on methods to deal with such behavior, which included contacting responsible adults and deescalating the situation, the situation settled down. Another patient, who was 16 at the time, was assaulted by a group of several teens while walking home from school. After the attack, he decided either to walk with friends or take a different route.

Let's look at several threatening situations and propose ways to deal with potential violence.

Scene 1: Someone calls you a bastard.

    Your response: 1. Speak to the perpetrator in a way that does not allow an escalation of the encounter, or

        2. Walk away from the situation.

Scene 2: An individual you don't like gets too close to you in order to provoke a confrontation.

    Your response: 1. Move away so that you will not be cornered, or

        2. Keep a leg in front of you as a barrier, or

        3. Walk away from the situation.

Scene 3: You are punched by someone you know.

    Your response: 1. Do not escalate the situation by returning verbal violence.

        2. If you have a weapon, do not use it.

        3. Remember that you don't need to be a winner or loser. Try to break even. If you humiliate the other person

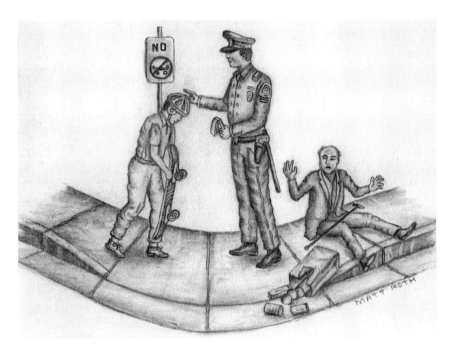

Be careful to control your emotions during stressful times.

or he humiliates you, then you might face even worse confrontations with him in the future.

Scene 4: Someone pulls out a weapon and points it at you.

> Your response:
> 1. Difficult though it may be, try to stay as calm as possible.
> 2. Attempt to defuse the situation by talking to the individual.
> 3. Do not act aggressively toward your potential assailant, and do not run unless you are fairly certain that it is safe to do so.
> 4. If money or valuables are the motive for the stickup, hand them over.
> 5. Lessen the tension any way you can.

Regrettably, during your adolescence, you may encounter many occasions for violent acts. Try to stay cool and levelheaded, and you should come out a winner.

DIVORCE

Two of my patients, both teens in the same family, were confronted with separation and divorce when their father left their mother and began a relationship with another woman. The younger boy was 13, and the older was 17, just on the verge of applying to college. Suddenly thrust into this situation, the younger boy withdrew from everyone except his mother. Although the older teen was stoic, he developed severe abdominal pains. About a year after the separation, both boys' symptoms began to improve. The younger one was helped by a counselor, and both boys continued a relationship with their father.

About 50 percent of marriages now end in divorce. Divorce stresses teens because of conflict between the parents, the loss of family stability, the loss of contact with one parent, economic hardships, and other factors. You have a right to feel angry, sad, embarrassed, and frightened if your parents separate and divorce each other. These feelings are expected and normal, and expressing them will probably help you in the long-term adjustment process.

Try venting your feelings to someone you can trust—a medical or psychological professional, a friend, an unrelated adult such as a teacher, relative, or another acquaintance. You can also find many resources on the Internet, such as the Children of Separation and Divorce Center, Inc. (*http./:shcosd.bayside.net/about.htm*).

DEATH

To this day, the pain associated with my father's sudden and unexpected death during my mid-adolescence seems fresh in my mind. The loss of a parent or friend without warning is exquisitely difficult, and the knowledge that the relationship will not continue into the future is terribly sad. In my case, we were also faced with financial problems. Eventually, we sold our home and moved to a smaller place. But I was more fortunate that others. I was quite close to my father's brother, my Uncle Joe. I believe that relationship helped me to survive my father's death emotionally intact. I developed coping skills; my life's work continued. Eventually, I found, the acute sadness mellows. But the sense of loss remains for decades. To help me deal with my father's death, I channeled emotional energy into my school work and research studies. Others may concentrate on athletics or relationships. A period of mourning is natural, as the wounds heal, your energy is focused on other areas. Do not let your feelings of grief manifest themselves in risky behaviors.

If a relative or friend has been profoundly ill for an extended period of time, death may come as a relief. Although you will also be sad, you may experience a sense that at least the person's endless pain and suffering are over. Communicating your feelings in words, art, or some other type of expressive medium may help you come to grips with the loss.

Several of my patients have lost close friends in accidents or suicides. Many male teens feel that nothing horrible can ever happen to them, that they are invincible. But the death of a peer is a stunning reminder of the fragility of life. Responding to such tragedies with reckless behavior is clearly inappropriate. Following the Littleton, Colorado, tragedy, there were many eulogies and memorials. Such a positive flow of emotional energy was useful to the families who lost loved ones and to the members of the community who grieved.

BREAKING UP WITH A LOVER

A natural part of adolescent development involves building relationships with others, becoming intimate in a variety of ways, and eventually ending many of these relationships. Of course, you may not be the one who ends the relationship. The other person might decide that it is over. Nevertheless, whenever a relationship ends, you are sad and feel a sense of loss.

Since male teens usually have a number of romantic relationships, they may experience a number of breakups. Generally, it is far easier to recover from a breakup than from a divorce or a death. The short-term feelings may be intense, but your coping mechanisms will alleviate the pain and unhappiness and, more likely, you will go on to develop another relationship. Channeling your emotional energies into other relationships, athletics, academics, or hobbies will help you heal faster.

LEAVING HOME

Ultimately, most teens leave home. If you attend a boarding school, you leave at an earlier age. If you don't, you may leave to attend college, to enroll in professional school, to enlist in the military, or, simply to live apart from your family. This is a normal rite of passage for American youth.

Since some of the adolescent developmental milestones have not been passed by the mid-teen years, leaving home for boarding school at age 14 or 15 is more difficult than leaving for college. On the other hand, most boarding-school faculty and staff are trained to deal with separation issues, including homesickness, insecurity, and sadness, which usually recede within a month or so. By the time teens are 17 or 18, the separation for college is easier. The urge for independence is strong, peer relationships are supportive, and you are ready to go. Many of the teens I see the summer before they enter college are very eager to leave home.

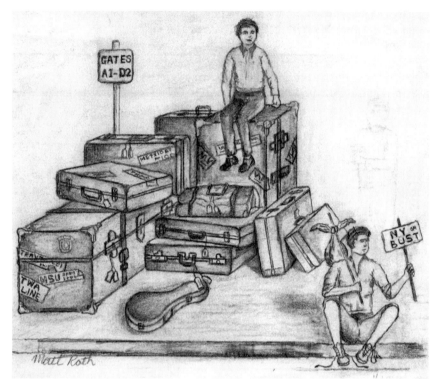

Leaving home is a normal rite of passage for American youth. Typically, separation issues, including homesickness, insecurity, and sadness, usually recede
within a month or so.

In fact, after they do enter college, I rarely hear any regrets or stories
about homesickness. The best advice is to keep in touch with your family. Most boys enjoy coming home during college breaks to eat delicious
food, have their laundry done by someone else, and sleep late.

REFERENCE

"Advice for Travelers." *The Medical Letter* 41 (April 23, 1999): 39–42.

Brown, Robert T., and Barbara A. Cromer, editors. *Psychosocial Issues in Adoles-
    cents, Adolescent Medicine: State of the Art Reviews*. Philadelphia: Hanley &
    Belfus, February, 1992.

Collipp, P. J., S. Goldzier, N. Weiss, et al. "Pyridoxine Treatment of Childhood
    Bronchial Asthma." *Annals of Allergy* 35 (1975): 93, 97.

Field, T., T. Henteleff, M. Hernandez-Reif, et al. "Children with Asthma Have
    Improved Pulmonary Functions After Massage Therapy." *Journal of Pedi-
    atrics* 132 (1998) 854–858.

Friedman, Standford B., and David R. DeMaso, editors. *Adolescent Psychiatric and Behavioral Disorders, Adolescent Medicine: State of the Art Reviews*. Philadelphia: Henley & Belfus, June 1998.

Fung, K. P., O. K. Chow, and S. Y. So. "Attention of Exercise-Induced Asthma by Acupuncture." *Lancet* 2 (1986): 1419–1422.

Kemper, Kathi J., and Mitchell R. Lester. "Alternative Asthma Therapies: An Evidence-Based Review." *Contemporary Pediatrics* 16 (March 1999) 3: 162–195.

McAnarney, Elizabeth, Richard Kreipe, Donald Orr, and George Comerci, editors. *Textbook of Adolescent Medicine*. Philadelphia: W. B Saunders Company, 1992.

Rich, Michael. "Pediatricians Should Educate Parents, Youths about Media's Effects." *AAP News* (September 1999): 28.

Strasburger, Victor C., and Donald E. Greydanus, editors. *The At-Risk Adolescent, Adolescent Medicine: State of the Art Reviews*. Philadelphia: Henley & Belfus, February 1990.

Vedanthan, P. K., L. K. Kesavalu, K. C. Murthy, et al. "Clinical Study of Yoga Techniques in University Students with Asthma: A Controlled Study." *Allergy Asthma Proc* 19 (1998) 1: 3.

Wacker, von A. "Healing in Asthma. A Pilot Study." *Erfahrungsheilkunde* (July 1996): 428.

11

Behavior, Mental and Emotional Health Issues

For many years, "storm and stress" were the terms used to characterize adolescents, assuming that adolescence was a period of emotional turmoil and mental-health disturbances. In fact, this is not true. Most male adolescents do not have any significant mental health problems. However, the frequency of certain mental conditions does increase during this period.

FOOD AND YOUR BEHAVIOR

I am certain that you have heard that teenage males act in bizarre ways because of their "strange" diets and eating habits. Does diet really influence behavior? Can you be harmed by too few or too many vitamins? How about sugar, food additives, caffeine, and skipping meals?

Deficiencies of niacin, water-soluble vitamins, thiamine, and pyridoxine may, indeed, lead to behavioral changes in adolescents. But nutritional deficiencies of these vitamins are exceedingly rare in the United States and would most likely occur in a teen with a chronic disease. Some males are iron deficient—though this condition is less common in males than females who have periodic menstrual blood loss. Studies on girls with iron-deficiency anemia have shown that, when they receive supplemental iron, they do better on certain tests of verbal learning and memory than girls with the same deficiency who did not receive iron. Since boys are less likely to be iron deficient, supplemental iron generally is not needed. And excessive iron in the body may be harmful.

Many parents and teachers insist that teens who eat lots of refined sugar have behavior problems, such as irritability and hyperactivity. Research studies have not been able to document this contention. Though the literature is filled with stories about food additives causing hyperactivity and learning disorders, most of the research has shown no relationship between artificial additives and behavior.

Teens generally like to spend time at coffee houses, and they drink lots of colas and other soft drinks. As a result, they consume significant amounts of caffeine. Too much caffeine may cause jitteriness and nervousness. While adolescent males may experience these symptoms after caffeine intake, there are no studies proving that behavior is strongly affected by the intake of a moderate amount of caffeine.

Are you one of the 20 percent of male adolescents who skip breakfast? Does skipping breakfast affect your school performance? Research on this is inconclusive. Although no link has been definitively established between skipping breakfast and poor academic performance, the lack of breakfast may indeed impair morning memory. Try to eat breakfast, especially before an important test or examination.

MENTAL HEALTH CONCERNS

Depression

A 16-year-old male came to my office for a general physical examination. A straight-A student at a highly competitive high school, he had few friends. Most weekends, he stayed home studying. Though he was exhausted, he slept poorly. During our talk, he explained that he was upset by his parents incessant fighting. Moreover, he wanted to date, but the opportunity had yet to arise. He had been quite unhappy for months. I diagnosed depression and referred him to a psychiatrist.

There are several medical causes for depression in adolescents. These include problems with hormones, such as a low thyroid rate (hypothyroidism). Neurological problems, such as sleep disturbances, may lie at the root of adolescent depression as well. Adolescents with chronic illness, such as cystic fibrosis, may be subject to depression. Some medications, including steroids, neurological drugs, and a few antibiotics, cause depression as a side effect.

Depression may be triggered by a feeling of loss of personal worth and lower self-esteem. These may be a result of

- academic stress
- parental divorce or other family separations
- breakup of a relationship

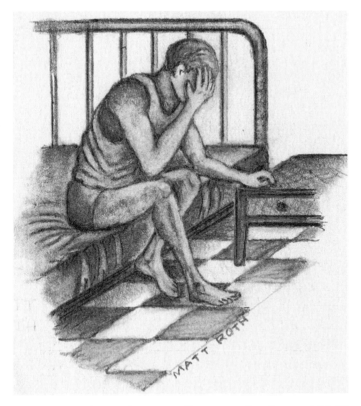

Studies have shown that up to 43 percent of males aged 14–15 may occasionally experience some symptoms of depression, such as feeling hopeless or persistently feeling empty or sad.

People who have unrealistic standards, lack effective coping skills, and feel that they do not receive sufficient love or support from the people who are important in their lives may also be at risk for depression.

Studies have shown that up to 43 percent of males age 14 to 15 may occasionally experience symptoms of depression. This does not mean that all these teens suffer from mental illness. In fact, most people have short periods when they feel depressed and are able to work through the symptoms themselves. This is not mental illness. Only a small percentage of adolescent males grapple with a clinical depression that could be classified as a mental illness.

As might be expected, genetics plays a role in depression (Jacobson and Rowe, 1999). Teens who have a parent or parents who are depressed are more likely to exhibit depressive symptoms. And in a study of college students with moderate to severe depression, it was found that they were more likely to have academic impairments, such as decreased academic productivity, increased absence from class, and more significant interpersonal problems, than their peers without depression (Heiligenstein et al., 1996).

Excellent medications, including a relatively new class of drugs, called selective serotonin reuptake inhibitors (SSRIs), are now available for depression. Serotonin is a neurotransmitter (a chemical substance that transmits nerve impulses) in the brain that regulates mood, activity, sleep patterns, and appetite. It is believed that depressive symptoms are more likely to occur in people with low levels of serotonin. The SSRI medications, including Prozac and Zoloft, boost the levels of serotonin at the cellular level in the brain. As a result, the levels of these neurotransmitters in the brain increase and the intensity of depressive symptoms usually decreases.

If you have some of the following symptoms of depression, you may wish to seek help:

• persistently feeling empty or sad
• feeling hopeless, pessimistic, guilty, or worthless
• loss of interest in ordinarily pleasurable activities, such as eating or exercising
• disturbances in sleep
• decreased energy
• persistent thoughts about death or suicide

If you think that a friend is depressed, you may be able to help by being a good listener. Be supportive of his or her feelings and be caring. If you have any sense that the situation may be serious, you should seek outside help.

Seasonal Affective Disorder (SAD)

Another 16-year-old patient started experiencing sadness, fatigue, and sleep difficulties each year in the late fall. His parents said that he was quite irritable and, at times, could not control his temper. He smashed his bedroom wall in a fit of anger. When I saw him that December, I learned that his father had been diagnosed with Seasonal Affective Disorder (SAD) and was using a light box several hours a day. A light box generates light which simulates sunlight. Patients with SAD sit in front of the light box and absorb the light by looking at the box. I referred the teenager to a psychiatrist, who diagnosed SAD. My patient was told to use a light box every morning. Gradually, his symptoms abated. In seasonal depression, which typically occurs during the months when there is less sunlight, patients develop signs of depression. Patients usually experience an improvement in the spring, when there is more sunlight.

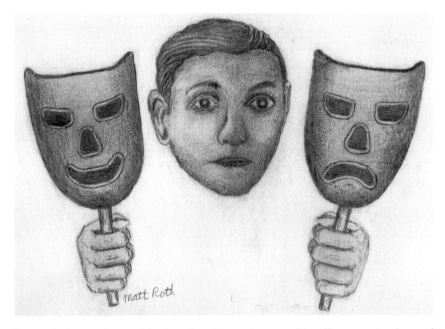

In manic depression, or bipolar disorder, patients could suffer a manic phase of elation, which, when untreated, may lead to depression.

If this pattern continues over a two-year period, it is labeled SAD. Understandably, SAD is more common in northern latitudes, when winter daylight is in shorter supply.

In a study of students at Bates College in Lewiston, Maine, 13 percent of the sample were found to have SAD. (Only 30 percent of the sample was male.) Patients with SAD apparently have disturbed body rhythms, caused by changes in the amount of sunlight they're exposed to. Studies in adults have found light boxes to be quite helpful.

Bipolar Disorder

I received a telephone call from a father who believed that his 19-year-old son was manic. The father said that his son rarely slept. He was also talkative and agitated. Over time, the young man's symptoms worsened, and the teen was referred to a psychiatrist who admitted him to a psychiatric facility. He responded well to lithium treatment.

In manic depression, or bipolar disorder, patients first suffer a manic phase of elation, euphoria, and sometimes, extreme irritability, which may lead to impairment in part because they cannot focus on a task. Untreated, the manic phase may lead to a depressive mood. According to the American Psychiatric Association, close relatives of people suffer-

ing from bipolar illness are 10 to 20 times more likely to develop depression or bipolar disorder.

Attention Deficit/Hyperactivity Disorder

A 14-year-old male came to see me because of failure in school. On
close review, it was apparent that he was not completing his school work
and homework, and he was having disciplinary problems in the class-
room. Further input from his parents and teachers indicated that he had
difficulty sustaining attention and could not concentrate on any one activity for more than a few minutes. Although these characteristics could
be traced back to his early years, he had managed to do sufficiently well
in school until ninth grade. In my office, he was jumpy and had poor
eye contact.

Following a consultation with a psychiatrist, the teen was diagnosed
with attention deficit/hyperactivity disorder (ADHD) and treated with
methylphenidate (Ritalin). His symptoms abated, and he began to succeed in school. It should be noted that attention deficit disorder (ADD)
is similar to ADHD; however, in ADD, the patient is not hyperactive.

ADHD and ADD are not uncommon in adolescents. Though the cause
of these disorders is not certain, some believe that it is biochemical in
origin. Fortunately, there are several good drug treatments. Some adolescents continue on medication through their college years into young
adulthood.

Post-traumatic Stress Disorder

Post-traumatic stress disorder (PTSD) may cause physical and behavioral problems in adolescents. In PTSD, the adolescent has a history of
a severe or terrifying physical or emotional event, ranging from sexual
abuse to personal violence, the sudden death of a friend or relative, or
seeing someone killed. The trauma from that experience may resurface
in the form of nightmares or flashbacks that make the adolescent feel as
if the original trauma were recurring. He may experience extreme emotional, physical, and mental distress when exposed to situations that re-
kindle memories of the original traumatic event. PTSD may also cause
sleep disturbances, problems in dealing with anger, and an inability to
concentrate. Symptoms of PTSD may appear as early as three months
after the original event or many years later. Adolescents who suffer from
PTSD should seek counseling.

Anxiety Disorders

Obsessive-Compulsive Disorder

Many of us have compulsive symptoms. To a certain extent, being
compulsive is beneficial. It is good practice to wear your seatbelt, to

check and recheck your written examinations, and to make sure that the gas stove is turned off. On the other hand, if you develop rituals—such as excessive hand washing, repeatedly opening and closing doors, and getting up and down from chairs—that become time consuming and interfere with normal functioning, then you may be suffering from an obsessive-compulsive disorder (OCD). An anxiety disorder, OCD may be disabling. The repetitive thoughts and behaviors may be senseless and extremely difficult to overcome.

I recall a boy who came to see me for a rash on his hands. He told me that he constantly washed his hands to rid them of "germs." I referred him to a psychiatrist who diagnosed OCD and prescribed medications. He is now free of symptoms. You should realize that some compulsive symptoms are perfectly normal. When these symptoms occur with signs of maladaptation and obsessive thoughts, however, then a diagnosis of OCD should be considered. Treatments may be quite effective.

Phobias

A phobia, another type of anxiety disorder, interferes with an individual's ability to go about his daily routine. Phobias occur when someone is presented with a feared object or dreaded situation. Phobic symptoms include profound fear, trembling, and panic. The following are some of the phobias that adolescent males may experience:

- fear of heights
- fear of school (school phobia)
- fear of public speaking
- fear of snakes, spiders, and stinging insects
- fear of closed spaces

While it is not well recognized, "school refusal" or school phobia, is a relatively common problem. Beginning in middle school, one of my patients developed vague illnesses, such as headaches, stomachaches, sore throats, and profound fatigue each year in September. These were never associated with fever, vomiting, diarrhea, or other objective signs of medical problems. While this pattern continued throughout most of the school year, he felt fine on weekends, vacations, and over the summer. He was diagnosed with school refusal.

School refusal may be related to other emotional concerns, seasonal affective disorder (SAD), problems at home, or behavioral issues. Your family, school, and medical providers may help you overcome this problem. My patient went on to graduate from high school. He is now in college and doing well.

In some cases, situations that trigger phobic symptoms may be avoided easily. Teens who have a fear of heights may decide not to climb mountains, and those who have a fear of snakes or spiders may stay away from them. But several of these phobias interfere with normal living. Since teens are required to attend school, at least until age 16, therapy is necessary for school phobia. Fear of public speaking may often be overcome with practice, and, sometimes, special courses.

In early adolescence, I had a violent reaction to a wasp sting. Since then, I have had an intense fear of wasps. When I see a wasp, I break out in a cold sweat and my heart races. I realize that this is an irrational fear. I have never undergone desensitization, which is the treatment for simple phobia. But I have talked about the problem with acquaintances. That has been helpful. I will now tolerate being in a room with a wasp. If it becomes necessary to kill the wasp, I defer to my wife.

Psychosomatic Illnesses

Some adolescent males develop physical symptoms caused by psychological factors. I remember the case of a 14-year-old boy in eighth grade who was transferred to a new school. Every day he had headaches. Frequently, he would visit the school nurse. Sometimes, his headaches would be so severe that he would be dismissed early from school. He told me that boys at school were bullying him. I determined that his anger, upset, and stress were causing these headaches. I suggested counseling, and he agreed. This is an example of a psychosomatic illness. Other psychosomatic symptoms include chest pain, abdominal pain, or altered bowel function. Treatment includes a good medical evaluation and counseling.

A 19-year-old saw me because of his inability to have an erection. He explained that although he had been able to have an erection with his previous partner, he was unable to do so with his current girlfriend. He mentioned that he did not drink alcohol before sex, which could contribute to the inability to obtain an erection. A complete physical examination was normal. During our conversation, he mentioned that he felt his girlfriend was overly aggressive with him. The relationship ended, and he became sexually active with another partner. In all but a very few cases, impotence in adolescence is due to psychological factors rather than a physical problem involving the genitalia or hormones. A sensitive and caring physician can help.

Suicide

Each year, there is about 1 suicide for every 10,000 teens. Suicide is more common among adolescent males, especially Caucasians. Teens who commit suicide often have a major mental illness such as depression. By itself, stress does not drive someone to suicide. The teenage victim of suicide frequently had no significant contact with medical or mental health providers. The teen may have suffered a loss of a crucial relationship, such as a relationship with a family member, lover, friend, or fellow athlete. The teen may feel pressure from his parents or rejection from his peers or parents. Most likely, he is depressed and may be abusing substances. Generally, there is a long-standing problem, and the suicide is triggered by a specific event. Teens who commit suicide usually have suicidal thoughts before they take action. These thoughts are followed by suicidal threats and attempts until, tragically, there is a successful suicide.

If you have suicidal thoughts, you must seek help. Most communities have a crisis intervention service that provides emergency counseling. Talk to your parents, siblings, relatives, teachers, guidance counselors, clergy, physician, and friends. They are all potential sources of assistance.

You may have a friend whom you believe is suicidal. If so, you should talk to this friend seriously and listen attentively. Express concern, acknowledge his or her feelings, and take action. Do not attempt to handle this problem yourself. Share your apprehensions with an adult and seek help from a professional.

The following are typical adolescent stressors that sometimes lead to suicidal thoughts or even suicide:

- changing relationships with parents
- hormonal changes
- peer pressure
- uncertainty about gender roles
- sexuality concerns
- parental marital discord
- problems in school

EMOTIONAL HEALTH

My father died suddenly and unexpectedly when I was 15. Needless to say, this was an extraordinarily stressful event in my adolescence. In addition to the loss of the love of my closest male relative, his death left the family with limited financial resources. My mother had to sell our home and move to an apartment. My dreams of attending a private college ended. How did I deal with this loss? I developed my own coping mechanisms. Since we had moved to a new neighborhood, I could no longer see some of my close friends. But I was able to continue at the same high school. My favorite uncle, who was kind and loving, began to play a greater role in my life. And I worked summers and received scholarship aid, which enabled me to attend the state university. Clearly, the road to become a physician was harder for me. Still, when one door closed, I found the way to open another.

Most people have to deal with stress in some form, and events that take place during adolescence may cause stress. Some of these are as follows:

- failing grades
- moving to a new home
- attending a new school
- death in the family
- serious illness in the family
- breakup with a girlfriend or lover
- sibling leaving home
- problems with police
- personal illness

Even under the most difficult circumstances, humans have the potential to adapt. Do not hesitate to turn to a counselor or your medical provider. They may be able to help you develop coping mechanisms. Basically, there are two main strategies for coping with emotional stressors. First, you need to learn to deal with a stressor without trying to change it. My father died; he was obviously not coming back. Since I could not change the stressor, I had to deal with the problem—my terrible sense of loss. Second, you must learn to focus on the issue. For example, if you receive a failing grade, you should speak to your teacher to arrange for extra assistance. By concentrating on your weaknesses in that subject, you, hopefully, will be able to improve your grade and remove that stressor.

Many of my patients have sleep disorders. They report that they are sleeping too much or too little and that their sleep is fitful and not refreshing. When they awaken, they are not rejuvenated. Instead, all too often, they wake up exhausted. Commonly, their problems are caused by a disturbance in their biological clock or circadian rhythm. Many teens do not realize that their body functions are rhythmic on a 24-hour basis controlled by a part of the brain. A common disturbance of the circadian rhythm occurs in jet lag, when one feels unwell after traveling through several time zones. Hormones associated with pubertal development cause adolescents to require more sleep than preadolescent children. Sleeping about eight hours a day is reasonable. However, social and/or academic pressures often keep teens up well past their usual bedtime. Many adolescents, who do not get sufficient sleep, develop a sleep debt. I had one patient who made up his sleep on weekends. He

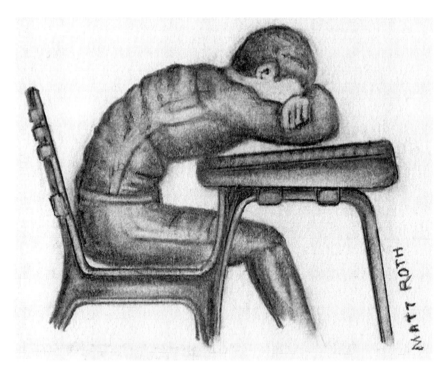

Hormones associated with pubertal development cause adolescents to require more sleep than preadolescent children. Getting insufficient sleep can lead to a sleep debt and excessive daytime sleepiness.

told me that one weekend he slept 26 hours without awakening. Of course, it is preferable to nap from time to time rather than to accumulate such a debt. You should know that if you stay up late for several nights in a row, you can alter your circadian rhythm. But, then, if you try to go to bed early, you may have difficulty falling asleep.

Sexual Abuse

Most adolescent males are reluctant to talk about sexual abuse and molestation. This is quite understandable. They fear disbelief by others, and, if they are abused by other males, they may feel threatened and embarrassed by the possible implications of homosexuality. It appears that preteen males are more likely to be abused by women. Most sexual abuse of males occurs within the family, up to 20 percent is perpetrated by people outside the family.

Some adult males are reluctant to talk about their past sexual abuse. Similarly, adolescent males may have a sense of shame, which is certainly unwarranted. They may also feel powerless. In spite of sexual abuse, most male victims do remarkably well emotionally as they enter adulthood. Studies of college males who had been abused seem to indicate that they do not experience long-term effects. There is little information that suggests that a history of male sexual abuse in childhood by other males causes the victim to become a homosexual. If you believe you have been abused, you should seek the help of a qualified counselor.

BEHAVIORAL PROBLEMS

Conduct Disorders

Are behavioral problems in adolescents a result of modern society or have these issues been present for centuries? In fact, the Bible refers to "incorrigible children." A child who killed his parent in the Roman Empire was put to death. Seventeenth-century Germany saw two teens executed for poisoning their uncle.

What are the warning signs for parents of adolescent males?

- Your son has friends who are in trouble with the law.
- You son gets into fights or has explosive outbursts.
- Your son is abusing alcohol.
- Your son has early or casual sex.
- Your son's school performance has been declining.
- Your son is missing school.

If your son exhibits one of the warning signs, it does not mean that he is headed for trouble. Yet, if he is demonstrating a pattern of misbehavior, he may have a conduct disorder. Conduct disorder (CD) is a psychiatric diagnosis. Some of its characterizing elements are:

- frequent lying
- forcing someone into sexual activity
- perpetrating acts of physical cruelty against others
- more than one episode of running away from home
- deliberately setting fires
- stealing on two or more occasions

Teens diagnosed with CD may also have an associated diagnosis, such as attention deficit disorder, substance abuse, depression, learning disabilities, and neurological abnormalities. These teens may also be from dysfunctional families. They require a thorough evaluation, including documentation of the problematic behaviors and the factors that contribute to them. Treatment may consist of the following:

- medication
- psychotherapy
- family therapy
- behavior modification
- parent training

Adolescent Violence

Adolescent violence is linked to poverty. Inner-city adolescent males are often poor and have high levels of unemployment. When the data are controlled for income, racial differences in homicide rates disappear or are significantly reduced. Plagued by poverty and unemployment, urban adolescent males are tempted to become involved in gang- and drug-related activities. These, in turn, lead to violence.

Gangs are a unified group of many individuals, usually predominately adolescent males. Some adolescents live, eat, and breath for their gangs. While the world in which they live may be frightening and impersonal, the gangs give male teens a sense of power, identity, prestige, security, and acceptance as well as protection from people who may threaten them. Membership in a gang serves as a means for an adolescent male to assert his independence from his family and formulate an identity apart from home in a new peer group. As you may recall, these are important goals of adolescent emotional growth and development. But gangs are extremely dangerous. They promote antisocial attitudes, including disregard for laws, schools, and family and other sources of authority. Moreover, violence permeates their everyday activities. And in the gang, new members often have their first sexual experiences with women and may start using illicit drugs.

Solutions to youth violence are complex, costly, and politically charged. At risk adolescents should be identified. Society must insist that more adolescents graduate from high school, obtain gainful employment, and live in suitable housing. Adult mentoring of potential gang members may decrease antisocial behavior and enhance academic achievement. Some researchers maintain that easy access to firearms causes youthful violence. Stronger antigun legislation and enforcement would undoubtedly cut down on violence committed by young people.

Adolescent violence may also be related to brain injuries. Under this theory, injury to the central nervous system, such as falls while riding a bicycle or head injuries from fights, makes people more likely to commit violent acts. However, this certainly does not provide a complete explanation for adolescent violence.

EDUCATIONAL ISSUES

The broad area of educational problems is beyond the scope of this book. Still, you can ask your physician for guidance if you are having an educational problem.

An 18-year-old patient who had already been accepted to a top university came to me for help. His handwriting was so illegible that his teachers could not read it. Since the essay readers undoubtedly would not be able to read his exam answers, he feared that he would not do well on the upcoming Advance Placement examinations. I asked him to give me a sample of his writing. Though I am able to read most types of writing, I was surprised that I could not read his. I suspected that he had a type of *dysgraphia*, or writing impairment. I sent him to a psychologist specializing in educational issues who certified the condition. The teen is now allowed to take examinations with a computer and printer.

There are other disabilities that may lead to educational problems in adolescents. After reading a story, an adolescent with a *sequencing disability* will not be able to recount the story in the proper sequence. An adolescent with an *abstraction disability* will not be able to understand the full meaning of abstract words, sentences, or paragraphs. He may not laugh at jokes because he does not understand them. Adolescents may also have a *short-term memory disability*. After reading or hearing material, teens with such disabilities will recall very little. Usually young people do not have both reading and auditory short-term memory disabilities together, and these teens often have normal long-term memory.

Adolescent males are largely resilient psychologically. The "storm and stress" of adolescence does not necessarily lead to or cause mental difficulties. All adolescents encounter stressful events and some emotional turmoil. Nonetheless, the vast majority of males make it through adolescence emotionally healthy. A single traumatic event should not lead to suicide; an emotional flare-up should not, in itself, be pathological; and everyone may experience periods of depression and euphoria. You need to be sensitive to your own feelings and those of your peers and be willing to seek help for yourself or your friends, should that be necessary.

You may feel that your parents are overly critical of you—sometimes too negative or too prone to give advice and issue orders. This is especially painful when you are hurting emotionally. Ask your parents to listen to you and your problems. Do not be afraid to ask others, such as your physician or school counselor, to help you open a dialogue with your parents. Much may be accomplished with the assistance of a third party.

RESOURCES

Hotlines and Web sites

American Academy of Child and Adolescent Psychiatry

Serves to aid in the understanding and treatment of developmental, behavioral, and mental disorders which affect children and adolescents.

http://www.aacap.org/web/aacap/info families/index.htm

1–800–333–7636

National Attention Deficit Disorder Association

Serves individuals with ADD; web site has section for teens.

http://www.add.org

1–800–487–2282

National Clearinghouse on Child Abuse and Neglect

A resource for professionals seeking information on the prevention, identification, and treatment of child abuse, neglect, and related child welfare issues.

http://www.calib.com/nccanch/

1–800–394–3366

National Institute on Drug Abuse

Information on drugs, treatment for addiction, and much more.

http://www.nida.nih.gov/NIDAHome1.html

National Institute of Mental Health

Information on many mental health disorders, including anxiety, depression, posttraumatic stress disorder, obsessive-compulsive disorder, learning disabilities, and phobias.

http://www.nimh.nih.gov/

1–800–421–4211

National Mental Health Consumer Self Help Clearinghouse

A resource for mental health consumers to improve their lives through self-help and advocacy.

http://www.mhselfhelp.org/

1–800–553–4539

National Runaway Switchboard

Offers crisis information, connection to families while teen is on the run; also provides free transportation for teen to return home.

1–800–621–4000

National Substance Abuse Helpline

A resource for teens to contact for assistance in obtaining help for drug abuse.

1–800–378–4435

Victims of Incest Can Emerge Survivors (VOICES)

A resource that assists victims of incest and child sexual abuse in becoming
survivors and to generate public awareness about the prevalence of incest.

http://www.voices-action.org/

1–800–786–4238

Books

Bancroft, John, and June Reinisch, editors. *Adolescence and Puberty*. New York:
Oxford University Press, 1990.

Brown, Robert T., and Barbara A. Cromer, editors. *Psychosocial Issues in Adolescents, Adolescent Medicine: State of the Art Reviews*. Philadelphia: Hanley &
Belfus, February, 1997.

Friedman, Stanford B., and David R. DeMaso, editors. *Adolescent Psychiatric and
Behavioral Disorders, Adolescent Medicine*. Philadelphia: Hanley & Belfus,
June 1998.

Friedman, Stanford B., Martin Fisher, and S. Kenneth Schonberg, editors. *Comprehensive Adolescent Health Care*. St. Louis: Quality Medical Publications,
Inc., 1992.

McAnarney, Elizabeth R., Richard E. Kreipe, Donald P. Orr, and George D. Comerci, editors. *Textbook of Adolescent Medicine*. Philadelphia: W. B. Saunders
Co., 1992.

Schydlower, Manuel, and Peter D. Rogers, editors. *Adolescent Substance Abuse and
Addictions, Adolescent Medicine: State of the Art Reviews*. Philadelphia: Hanley & Belfus, June 1993.

Strasburger, Victor C., and Donald E. Greydanus. *The At-Risk Adolescent, Adolescent Medicine: State of the Art Reviews*. Philadelphia: Hanley & Belfus, February 1990.

Wiener, Jerry M., editor. *Textbook of Child & Adolescent Psychiatry*. 2nd Edition.
Washington, D.C.: American Psychiatric Press, 1997.

Articles

Jacobson, K., and D. Rowe. "Genetic and Environmental Influences on the Relationships between Family Connectedness, School Connectedness and
Adolescent Depressed Mood: Sex Differences." *Developmental Psychology*
35 (July 1999) 4: 926–939.

Heiligenstein, E., G. Guenther, K. Hsu, and K. Herman. "Depression and Academic Impairment in College Students." *Journal of American College Health*
45 (September 1996) 2: 59–64.

Health and Medicine Search Engines

Alcohol, *http://achoo.com*

Health A to Z *http://www.healthatoz.com*

Health Web Sites

Medical Literature, *http.//www.nlm.nih.gov*

U.S. Government, *http:www.healthfinder.gov*

Magazines

Heilgenstein, E., G. Guenther, K. Hsu, and K. Herman. "Depression and Academic Impairment in College Students." *Journal of American College Health* 4 (February 1996) 2: 59–64.

Low, K. G., and J. M. Feissner. "Seasonal Affective Disorder in College Students: Prevalence and Latitude." *Journal of American College Health* 47 (March 1998) 3: 135–137.

Pamphlets

"Anxiety Disorders." Washington, D.C.: American Psychiatric Association, 1997.

"Dealing with Depression: What Everyone Should Know." Baltimore, Md.: American College Health Association, 1996.

"Depression." Washington, D.C.: American Psychiatric Association, 1997.

Greydanus, Donald E., and Helen D. Pratt. "Emotional and Behavioral Disorders of Adolescence: Part 1, Adolescent Health Update." *American Academy of Pediatrics* 7(1995) 3: 1–8

"If You Suspect Someone You Care about Is Considering Suicide . . ." Chicago, Ill.: National Depressive and Manic-Depressive Association, 1992.

"Manic-Depressive/Bipolar Disorder." Washington, D.C.: American Psychiatric Association, 1993.

"Obsessive-Compulsive Disorder." Washington, D.C.: American Psychiatric Association, 1992.

"Obsessive-Compulsive Disorder." Bethesda, Md.: National Institute of Mental Health, 1996.

"Phobias." Washington, D.C.: American Psychiatric Association, 1992.

Ryan, Sheryl A. "Helping Parents Communicate with Their Teens: Adolescent Health Update." *American Academy of Pediatrics* 11(1999) 2: 1–8.

Spence, W. R. "Suicide Can Be Prevented." Waco, Tex.: HEALTH EDCO, 1992.

"Teen Depression and Suicide." Alexandria, Va.: National Mental Health Association, 1997.

Presentation

Dakker, Anthony, and Lena Kontz. "Violence in Youth: The Effects of Gangs." Presented at the Society for Adolescent Medicine meetings. Los Angeles: March 1999.

12

Cross-Cultural Issues and Your Health

At the millennium—the year 2000—approximately 40 percent of the U.S. population under the age of 19 were minorities. Since culture, race, ethnic group, poverty, and affluence all play important roles in health-related beliefs, behaviors, and access to optimal healthcare services, minorities may be faced with unique healthcare issues.

First, let's define some terms:

minority: A minority is a group of people who differ in race, religion, or culture from the majority of individuals. In the United States, African Americans and Hispanics are two of many minorities.

culture: A culture consists of a group's thoughts, communications, customs, beliefs, actions, values, and institutions. For example, the Hasidic sect of Orthodox Jews has its own culture.

race: A race is a population of people who have common physical characteristics. Asians and Caucasians are races.

ethnic group: A group of people who share a common and distinct culture, religion, and language. Gypsies are an ethnic group.

acculturation: Acculturation refers to the process of adopting the culture of the majority group.

Male adolescents from different cultures may have different concepts of health. For male teens in Mongolia, for example, survival is key. There, homeless adolescents live in sewers and scavenge for food. Urban Latinos have health concerns that are linked to the environment in which they live. These may include illnesses, such as asthma, which may be caused by poor air quality; conditions resulting from poverty, such as malnutrition and violence; and sexually transmitted disease. Affluent suburban white males may direct more of their attention to their appearance and worry about acne, hair loss, height, or even eating disorders.

Adolescent health behaviors vary by race. According to a national survey conducted by the Centers for Disease Control (CDC), 39 percent of white high school males recently engaged in binge drinking. That contrasted with the 25 percent of the African American high school students who reported such activity. Studies have shown that Asian adolescents drink less than whites, Native Americans, Hispanics, and African Americans. However, the amount of alcohol consumption among Asian teens increases with their acculturation into U.S. society. The longer an adolescent is in this country, the more likely it is that he will be acculturated.

In the CDC survey, 32 percent of white male teens were currently sexually active. That stands in sharp contrast to 58 percent of African American males, who report participating in sexual activity. When compared to white and African American males, Hispanic males are more likely to abstain from sex.

Healthcare-seeking practices may also vary by ethnic group. I recall caring for a Chinese student, born in Mainland China, who had recurrent headaches. Over time, it became apparent that he had a psychiatric problem. But his cultural background would not allow him to acknowledge mental illness. So, he subconsciously altered his symptoms to physical complaints that were more culturally acceptable. In China, mental problems are handled by family members within the family unit. On the Mainland, seeing a psychiatrist would not be considered an option.

But other groups also have strong health-related beliefs. Christian Scientists will not allow themselves or their children to receive blood transfusions. And when I was in practice near the Navajo reservation in New Mexico, I often had to combine my practice of medicine with the types of healing practiced by the Indian medicine man.

Some adolescent males, especially those who have recently immigrated to the United States, may have been raised in a family and culture in which views of disease are radically different from those in the U.S. mainstream. In her book *The Spirit Catches You and You Fall Down*, Anne Fadiman describes the story of a Hmong (Asian) child with a seizure disorder. While the child's parents believed that her seizures were caused by a wandering of her soul, American physicians maintained that they were due to a misfiring of the patient's brain cells. Misunderstandings between the family and the doctors led to a bad outcome. The child suffered severe seizures, which resulted in serious brain damage.

Latino cultures may use a "hot" or "cold" classification to describe illness, medications, or foods. According to Latino culture, in the body, there is a balance between hot and cold. Illness occurs when there is an imbalance. Thus, treatment includes consuming foods and/or herbs from the "opposite" group. For example, diarrhea is a hot disease. Therefore, it would be treated with a cold food such as bananas. A respiratory "cold" infection is a cold disease. So a hot medication, such as aspirin, may be given. While Western medicine would recommend plenty of cold juices for a person with a respiratory cold, this advice would probably be ignored by someone who believes in the hot/cold theory. Instead, that person would favor hot foods such as chili peppers, onions, or garlic.

Teens who are new to the United States may experience symptoms of culture shock. The food, climate, and even some germs may be unfamiliar. As a result, they may feel unwell. Generally, this is a temporary condition.

If you are from another culture or ethnic group, it is vitally important to communicate effectively with your healthcare provider, which may be a challenge if you do not speak English well. Nevertheless, you should attempt the following:

• Describe your medical problem as you understand it and in your own words.
• Tell your healthcare provider what you think is causing your illness, even if it sounds ridiculous.
• Try to convey when and why the problem started. For example, you might say, "I developed a cold after I went outside with wet hair."
• Tell your healthcare provider what you think may help you get better.

Cross-cultural issues also affect how you access the U.S. healthcare system. The United States has no national health insurance. So either you or your insurer—or both—pay for your healthcare. If you are an immigrant who is poor, you may be unable to pay for healthcare. As a result, you will have less access to healthcare. And you may be unfamiliar with nurse-practitioners, who fill an important mid-level role in U.S. healthcare. In your native country, there may be no nurse-practitioners.

You should know that healthcare providers are not necessarily trained in issues common to other cultures, ethnic groups, or races. And you may know little about the background of your healthcare provider. Since it is important for your personal medical care to be optimal, you should convey your cultural beliefs when you seek care. If your provider is sensitive and caring, he or she will take the time to answer your questions.

REFERENCES

Bancroft, John, and June Reinisch, editors. *Adolescence and Puberty*. New York: Oxford University Press, 1990.

Fadiman, Anne. *The Spirit Catches You and You Fall Down*. New York: Farrar, Straus, and Giroux, 1997.

Fisher, Martin, Linda Juszczak, and Lorraine Klerman, editors. *Prevention Issues in Adolescent Health Care, Adolescent Medicine: State of the Art Reviews*. Philadelphia: Henley & Belfus, February 1999.

Friedman, Stanford, and David DeMaso, editors. *Adolescent Psychiatric and Behavioral Disorders, Adolescent Medicine: State of the Art Reviews*. Philadelphia: Henley & Belfus, June, 1998.

Helman, Cecil. *Culture, Health and Illness*. London: Wright, 1990.

McAnarney, Elizabeth, Richard Kreipe, Donald Orr, and George Comerci, editors. *The Textbook of Adolescent Medicine*. Philadelphia: W. B. Saunders, 1992.

13

Issues for Gay Adolescents

In October 1998, following a brutal beating, Matthew Shepard, a 21-year-old gay college student, died. The beating was attributed to antigay violence, and several individuals were charged with his murder.

The incident precipitated national demonstrations, and there was a candlelight vigil on the steps of the Capitol in Washington. Violence is one of several issues gay adolescents may face as they go through adolescence. The Matthew Shepard murder is an extreme and, fortunately, very rare example of antigay violence.

First we need to define some terms:

gay: For the purposes of this chapter, *gay* refers to males with a homosexual orientation.

gender identity: This is your personal sense of being either a male or female. Gender identity is established early in life.

sexual orientation: This refers to your physical behavior toward and emotional/erotic attraction to others. Homosexuality is a same-sex attraction; bisexuality is attraction to both sexes; heterosexuality is attraction to the opposite sex.

sex roles: These are social and cultural attitudes and stereotypes of male and female behaviors, which are usually established between ages 3 and 7.

in the closet: The condition of a gay person who poses as a heterosexual and is unwilling to publicly disclose his sexual orientation.

coming out: This is your personal recognition that you have same-sex feelings and additionally it is also when you inform others that you are gay.

antigay violence: This is violence and crimes against gays that are related to bias and prejudice.

It has been estimated that between 5 percent and 10 percent of all males are gay. Gay people are found in all ethnic groups, races, religions, socioeconomic classes, backgrounds, and nationalities. Gay males are successful athletes, doctors, teachers, artists, blue-collar workers, writers, and members of other professions, trades, or businesses. Years ago, being gay was classified as a disease. For decades, we have known that this is not true although there are some who mistakenly believe that it is a disease. Given the love and support that all of us should receive, gay males are just as likely to develop into happy, healthy, and successful adults as heterosexual males.

According to Richard R. Troiden, gay identity development occurs in four stages, over a period of time, as noted below:

Stage I—Sensitization. This occurs before the onset of pubertal development. Gay males may feel different from their peers. Yet, they do not perceive themselves to be sexually different.

Stage II—Identity Confusion. Generally, after the onset of puberty, gay adolescents become aware of same-sex thoughts. These teens are confused, often closeted, and they usually develop coping skills.

Stage III—Identity Assumption. Between the ages of 15 and 21, some gay adolescents self-identify and come out, especially to their gay peers. Often, as they gain access to organized gay communities, their self-image improves.

Stage IV—Commitment. In this state, which usually occurs in adulthood, the gay male incorporates his sexual identity into many or all aspects of life. His sexual identity is shared with nongay friends and family members.

Gay adolescents must develop coping mechanisms to deal with societal perceptions, attitudes, and prejudices against gays. Unfortunately, many members of society mistakenly feel that gays are unhappy, even mentally ill, and cannot have long-term relationships. The senseless murder of Matthew Shepard dramatically demonstrated that gay adolescents may be hated, feared, and pitied for absolutely no reason. Sometimes, only because they are gay, gay adolescents have been the target of hate crimes, discrimination, ridicule, harassment, and violence. Hopefully, as more gay males come out and share their lives with friends, family, colleagues, and one another, we will see a reduction in these serious problems.

With so much negative energy directed at gay males, it is especially challenging for them to develop a positive self-identity. But adolescents should develop such a self-identity. The entire process may be facilitated by coping mechanisms and social support. Coping mechanisms include trying to find supportive individuals, programs, or communities. For example, a gay male may prefer to live in a community that is supportive of gay individuals rather than antigay. Social clubs and other organiza-

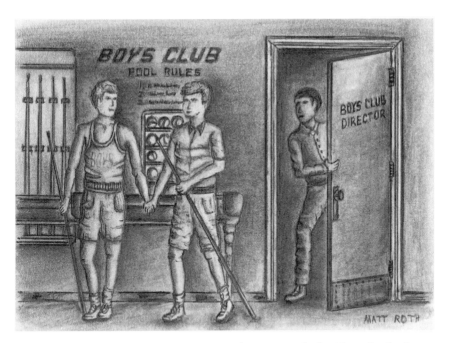

Gay adolescents must develop coping mechanisms to deal with societal misperceptions, negative attitudes, and prejudices against gays.

tions may help gays meet one another in safe circumstances. A supportive family, peers, and adults also help a gay adolescent develop a positive self-identity. And, finally, positive adult role models and gay community resources may be very helpful to a gay teen struggling with identity issues. Of course, a supportive physician and other healthcare practitioners are of equal importance.

HEALTHCARE CONCERNS

The health issues of gay teens are not necessarily any different from those of straight teens. But they may have a higher incidence of certain medical or mental health issues.

Much like heterosexual males, gay males are subject to sexually transmitted diseases (STDs). These STDs include HIV, syphilis, genital warts, herpes, gonorrhea, hepatitis A, hepatitis B, chlamydia, lice, and scabies. (For more details on sexually transmitted diseases, see Chapter 5, "Sexuality.") The difference is that certain STDs are more common among gay males. Specifically, HIV has always been more prevalent in gay adolescent males than in straight adolescent males in the United States.

Forty-nine percent of the males in Massachusetts who have been diagnosed with AIDS are males who have sex with other males.

Gay adolescent males report that they use sexual experiences to learn about being gay. These experiences are likely to include unprotected anal intercourse. However, because the mucosa or skin of the anus is thin and easily torn, it is particularly risky for a gay male to be the recipient of unprotected anal intercourse. Due to the friction of intercourse, it is more likely that organisms such as HIV can penetrate the mucosa of the anus and lead to an infection. (This type of intercourse is called anal receptive.) Always practice safe sex and use condoms during intercourse.

Because of societal prejudices and attitudes, it may be difficult for gay adolescents to meet and socialize with other gay adolescents. I recall two patients, one 16 and the other 17, who had sexual experiences with gay males that they regretted. The first patient was closeted and just coming to terms with his sexual orientation. On the Internet, he established a relationship with a gay male. After a period of correspondence on the Internet, they arranged to meet. My patient had consensual but unprotected receptive intercourse. After it was over, he was quite upset. The second patient knew a gay male at his workplace. They met at the other male's home. My patient was forced to have nonconsensual, anal receptive intercourse, which was frightening and humiliating to him. Both patients were placed at high risk for sexually transmitted disease by these actions.

There are no convincing data demonstrating that gay adolescents use substances such as alcohol or drugs more or less than straight adolescents. Gay and straight teens use substances for many of the same reasons: experimentation, assertion of independence, relief of stress, increasing feelings of self-esteem, or self-medication for problems such as depression. Because of societal attitudes and biases, as well as their confusion about sexual orientation, gay adolescent males may lack self-esteem, and, as a result, may be tempted to try illegal drugs.

MENTAL HEALTH CONCERNS

Teens who believe they are gay, or who accept that they are gay, are faced with enormous challenges. Intolerance may result in rejection by family members, peers, teachers, coaches, and other important people in their lives. These psychological issues place them at greater risk for mental health problems. Gay adolescents are more likely to suffer from depression and/or commit suicide than are their straight peers. One government study found that gay adolescents attempted suicide two to three times more often than heterosexual adolescents. Thirty percent of gay and bisexual male adolescents have attempted suicide at least one time. Many gay males between the ages of 15 and 19 have sought mental health services. If you feel depressed or suicidal, seek the services of a physician or a therapist and tell your family.

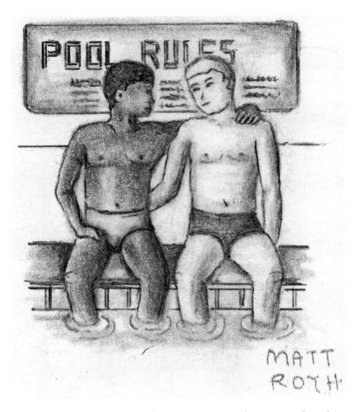

Teens who either believe they are gay or who accept that they
are gay are often faced with enormous challenges.

Gay adolescents and young adults have mental health concerns related
to their sexual orientation, as noted in the following chart:

Concern	Prevalence in Gay Males Ages 18–25 Years
Coming out to parents	93%
Coming out to friends	63%
Relationship with family	60%
Sadness/depression	63%
Anxiety	77%
Concerns about AIDS	92%
Alcohol use	22%
Drug use	18%

Source: D'Augelli (1991).

For the most part, gay teens are typical adolescents from typical families living typical lives. They have not chosen to be gay, and their upbringing did not make them gay. In all probability, gay sexual orientation has both a biological and an environmental basis. In 1991, J. Michael Bailey, Ph.D., and his associates conducted an interesting study on gay men and their identical and fraternal twins as well as their adoptive brothers. (Identical twins have the same genetic makeup; fraternal twins have a different genetic makeup. And adoptive brothers have no common genes with their brothers.) Fifty-two percent of the identical twins of the gay men were gay. On the other hand, only 22 percent of the fraternal twins of the gay men were gay. These data are consistent with the strong influence that biology or genes have on sexual orientation for males. Adoptive brothers of gay men were gay in 11 percent of the cases. This finding suggests there is a more limited role for environment in determining sexual orientation. Furthermore, it demonstrates that there are at least several influences on male sexual identity, with biology being a powerful one and environment being secondary, but still important. There may also be other influences as well.

Since coming out has so many risks, gay adolescents often remain in the closet. But coming out is part of the normal development of the gay adolescent as he approaches the end of adolescence. Coming out may, in itself, help relieve some of the stressors related to sexual orientation and promote a heathier and happier life.

REFERENCES

Bailey, J. Michael, and Richard C. Pillard. "A Genetic Study of Male Sexual Orientation." *Archives of General Psychiatry* 48 (December 1991): 1089–1096.
Council on Scientific Affairs. "Health Care Needs of Gay Men and Lesbians in the United States." *Journal of the American Medical Association* 275 (1996): 1354–1359.
D'Augelli, A. "Gay Men in College: Identity Processes and Adaptations. *Journal of College Student Development* 30 (1991): 140.
Greydanus, Donald, Kimball Miller, and Helen Pratt, editors. *Frontiers of Academic Medicine and Health Care Delivery in the 1990s, Adolescent Medicine: State of the Art Reviews*. Philadelphia: Hanley & Belfus, October 1994.
Massachusetts Department of Public Health. "Massachusetts HIV/AIDS Quarterly Review" (May 1999).
Pillard, Richard C., and J. Michael Bailey. "A Biologic Perspective on Sexual Orientation." *The Psychiatric Clinics of North America* 18 (March 1995) 18: 71–84.
Pollack, William. *Real Boys*. New York: Random House, 1998.
Ryan, Caitlin, and Donna Futterman, editors. *Lesbian and Gay Youth: Care and Counseling, Adolescent Medicine: State of the Art Reviews*. Philadelphia: Hanley & Belfus, June 1997.

RESOURCES

Advocacy Organizations

National Gay and Lesbian Task Force (NGLTF)
1734 14th Street, NW
Washington, DC 20009–4309
202–332–6483
202–332–0207 (fax)
http://www.ngltf.org

Sexual Information and Educational Council of the U.S. (SIECUS)
130 West 42nd Street, Suite 2500
New York, NY 10036
212–819–9770
http:/; shwww.siecus.org

Dignity USA
1500 Massachusetts Ave., NW, No. 11
Washington, DC 20005
800–877–8797
http:/; shwww.dignityusa.org

National Youth Advocacy Coalition
1711 Connecticut Avenues, NW, Suite 206
Washington, DC 20009
202–319–7596

Service Agencies for Gay Youth

Sidney Borum Jr. Health Center
130 Boylston Street
Boston, MA 02116
617–457–8150

Health Initiatives for Youth, Inc. (HIFY)
1242 Market Street
San Francisco, CA 94102
415–487–5777
415–487–5771 (fax)
http://www.hify.com

Horizons Community Services
Youth Services & Anti-Violence Program

961 West Montana Street

Chicago, IL 60614–2408

773–472–6469

773–929-HELP (helpline)

773–871-CARE (Anti-Violence Project, 24 hour crisis hotline)

http://www.qrd.org/qrd/www/usa/illinois/horizons/horizons.html

Evelyn Hooker Center for Gay and Lesbian Mental Health

Department of Psychiatry

The University of Chicago

5841 South Maryland Avenue (MC3077)

Chicago, Illinois 60637–1470

773–702–9725

Boston HAPPENS Program

Division of Adolescent Medicine

The Children's Hospital

300 Longwood Avenue

Boston, MA 02115

617–355–8496

http://web1.tch.harvard.edu/adolescent/happens/contact.html

Books

Borhek, Mary V. *Coming Out to Parents: A Two-Way Survival Guide for Lesbians and Gay Men and Their Parents*. Cleveland: The Pilgrim Press, 1993.

Due, Linnea A. *Joining the Tribe: Growing Up Gay and Lesbian in the '90s*. New York: Anchor Books, 1995.

Rench, Janice E. *Understanding Sexual Identity: A Book for Gay and Lesbian Teens*. Minneapolis: Lerner Publications, 1990.

Singer, Bennett L., editor. *Growing Up Gay: A Literary Anthology*. New York: Free Press, 1993.

Whitlock, Katherine. *Bridges of Respect: Creating Support for Lesbian and Gay Youth*. Philadelphia: American Friends Service Committee, 1989.

14

Chronic Conditions

During the summer of 1999, Lance Armstrong, a 27-year-old bicyclist, became only the second American to win the Tour de France, a grueling 2,286-mile, 21-day road race in France. By anyone's measure, that would be an extraordinary accomplishment.

But there is more to Armstrong's story than winning the Tour de France. In 1996, he was diagnosed with testicular cancer that had spread to his lungs, abdomen, and brain. In addition to surgery to remove the cancerous testicle, Armstrong underwent chemotherapy. Many people were convinced that his years of competitive cycling were over.

Armstrong, however, would not let his chronic illness stand in the way of his dreams. Even during his cancer treatments, he rallied and began workouts to regain his strength and stamina. At times, Armstrong considered quitting. Battling cancer and preparing for a return to competitive cycling did not appear to be compatible goals. Still, he persevered. And on July 25, 1999, Armstrong triumphantly carried the U.S. flag around the Champs Elysees in Paris. A few months after the win, his wife gave birth to their first child.

Fortunately, cancer is relatively rare among adolescents. But there are other chronic conditions that do occur more frequently. In fact, according to Newacheck and McManus (1991) 31.5 percent of U.S. adolescents have one or more chronic conditions. According to Newacheck and McManus, the following are the most common chronic health conditions in individuals between the ages of 10 and 17:

Chronic Condition	Rate per 1,000 persons, ages 10–17 years
Respiratory Allergies	130.3
Asthma	46.8

Chronic Condition	Rate per 1,000 persons, ages 10–17 years
Frequent or Severe Headache	45.8
Eczema and Skin Allergies	35.2
Frequent or Repeated Ear Infections	33.6

A significant number of adolescents are physically challenged to a mild, moderate, or severe degree. Like other people, they benefit from exercise, which increases lung volume, cardiac output, and muscle mass. Hoping to encourage sports participation among those with physical limitations, the National Wheelchair Athletic Association was formed in 1957. The association has introduced those in wheelchairs to track and field, swimming, table tennis, archery, and weight lifting. The Boston Marathon, which is run every year in April, has wheelchair divisions for both men and women.

Male teens with chronic illness or disability may struggle with body-image issues. This is especially true as they go through the physical and developmental changes in puberty. Yet, it should not be assumed that they have any more mental health problems than teens without chronic conditions.

But, teens with chronic illnesses should be aware that their illness may have an impact on their education. After all, such teens may miss classes, exams, or field trips because of needed treatments. And, they may be forced to adapt. As a result of a teen accident, Matthew Roth, the person who illustrated this book, was paralyzed from his neck down. Since he could no longer write with his hands, he learned to write with a pencil in his mouth. Later in life, he realized that he could also use a pencil to draw.

To ensure that teachers and the school system are responsive to their special needs, teens with chronic illness often benefit from advocates. Matthew's parents and his siblings were always there to lend assistance.

And teens with chronic disease or disabilities may face discrimination on the job and difficulties in their sexual lives. Clearly, Lance Armstrong is a success story—an individual who beat overwhelming odds and disabilities. Even though his original Tour de France sponsor dropped him because they were skeptical of his ability to compete professionally, within months he announced his affiliation with the U.S. Postal Service pro cycling team. The following are the stories of some of my patients who have chronic conditions. All the names have been changed.

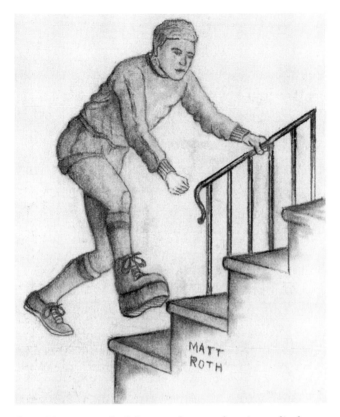

Over 30 percent of adolescents have a chronic medical condition.

OBESITY

I met Ralph, who is now 18 years old, about eight years ago. Four years ago, he told me that he was experiencing periods of depression that alternated with periods of hyperactivity. He was placed on Lithium, a medication that unfortunately brought on hypothyroidism, or a slowing of his thyroid, as a side effect. Subsequently, he developed problems with his school work, and, despite excellent control of his thyroid problem, he had a slow but steady weight gain.

Eventually, Ralph became 30 percent overweight for his height. During his early high school years, he had fluctuating moods. His parents decided that he would be better served at a different high school. And that proved to be true. At his new school, Ralph began to eat a healthier diet and to exercise. His academic record also improved markedly.

By his high school graduation, Ralph had lost 40 pounds. After a year

of traveling, he entered college. His weight remains well in proportion
to his height.

NEUROFIBROMATOSIS

I first saw Leonard when he was 12 years old. Immediately, I noted
that he had an unusual skin rash, and I worried that it might indicate a
serious illness.

Regrettably, my concerns were confirmed by a neurologist, and Leonard was diagnosed with neurofibromatosis, a lifelong disease in which
there is a skin rash and, sometimes, swollen bumps under the skin.
Linked to genetics, it may be transmitted to offspring.

Although he was very successful in high school, he was engaging in
some risky sexual behaviors. Leonard has since accepted his illness, stays
away from risky sex, and is excelling at a prestigious New England college.

LEARNING DISABILITIES

Samuel is a 14 year old who began to experience difficulties with his
school work in middle school. Problems occurred in math, spelling, and
writing compositions. An evaluation revealed that he had sequencing
difficulties. Following multistep directions was difficult. He was placed
in special education and has done remarkably well since.

Shortly after birth, Adam was adopted by a professional couple. In
middle school, Adam started misbehaving and he was doing poorly in
school. His grades were poor, and he was often sent to the principal's
office for disciplinary action.

At the time, Adam was evaluated by a neurologist who diagnosed
attention deficit disorder without hyperactivity. He was started on Ritalin, a medication that helped him focus on his work. Now in high
school, Adam is doing well in most of his subjects.

PHYSICAL DISABILITIES

Paul was born with a severely scarred cornea, which left one of his
eyes without any vision. When he was still a baby, the eye was surgically
removed, and it was replaced with a prosthesis. Over the years, as his
head grew, he received larger prostheses.

Although Paul was never permitted to play contact or collision sports,
he did become an outstanding cross-country runner. And he never allowed his disability to affect his school work or social life. He is now a
successful college student.

Patrick was born with weakness of his right arm and right leg. Despite these conditions, he learned to write using his right hand. His writing was illegible, and he received low grades because of this disability. When I learned of this problem, I referred him to an occupational therapist to improve the quality of his writing. With more legible writing, his grades are now better.

MAJOR DEPRESSION

I first met Michael when he was around 14 years old. His parents warned me that he did not like doctors, and he would not speak to them. After our first meeting, I diagnosed depression and referred Michael to a psychiatrist.

The psychiatrist determined that Michael required psychiatric hospitalization. For months, Michael received inpatient treatment. Following discharge, he had trouble adjusting to high school early on. Then he began to achieve academically. After high school, Michael attended a prestigious college, where he was a premedical student. Now Michael is attending medical school, and he plans to practice medicine.

CROHN'S DISEASE

George was a senior in high school when he developed bloody, crampy bowel movements. At that time, a former girlfriend was stalking him.

When he came to see me, he was thin for his height, anemic, and fatigued. Within a few weeks, he was diagnosed with Crohn's disease, an inflammatory bowel disease (IBD). George was placed on a number of medications including oral steroids. He enrolled in college, but left after the first semester. As he went from job to job, his IBD symptoms waxed and waned.

Eventually, George turned to medical providers who practiced complementary medicine. That seemed to trigger a desire in George to beat his problems, and he developed a positive attitude toward life, his body, his family, and his peers. In time, George stopped taking all his medications, and he continues to do well.

DIABETES

During his senior year of high school, Anthony began to lose weight, urinate excessively, and feel extremely fatigued. After a blood test showed that his blood sugar was very high, he was diagnosed with diabetes mellitus.

To help him learn about diabetes and how to manage his blood sugar, Anthony was hospitalized for a few days. Once his blood sugar was under control, he returned to athletics. Anthony is now an outstanding student athlete who attends a top college. His diabetes, which is a life-long illness, continues to be well controlled.

AIDS

Before testing for HIV was routinely performed, John acquired HIV from a blood transfusion. Several years later, he was diagnosed with full-blown AIDS, and he was placed on medications.

While he has occasionally needed hospitalizations for AIDS-related complications, John has maintained an outstanding academic record. A recent college graduate, John plans a career in scientific research. Of course, he continues to take medication.

CANCER

At the age of 19, shortly after completing his first year of college, Robert noticed a lump in his neck. Concerned, I referred him to a specialist who diagnosed non-Hodgkin's lymphoma, a form of cancer.

Since Robert did not respond well to chemotherapy, his oncologist advised a bone marrow transplant. The treatment made Robert quite ill and weak. And he was susceptible to infection. Still, he was able to finish college with his class. His lymphoma is now under excellent control, and he is beginning his career as an engineer.

RENAL FAILURE

About 10 years ago, when Thomas was a high school student, a lab test revealed that there was protein in his urine. I referred him to a kidney specialist who diagnosed focal glomerulosclerosis, a chronic kidney problem.

Regrettably, Thomas's kidney function quickly failed, and his kidneys stopped performing their blood-cleaning function. He was forced to begin renal dialysis, a technique in which blood is cleared of impurities, a necessary function usually accomplished by the kidneys. In spite of his medical problems and the many hours each week he spent on dialysis, Thomas did well academically and excelled in college and participated in sports. After a few years, he received a kidney transplant. Since then he has functioned extremely well.

Disabilities are very common in adolescents. With determination and perseverance, one can overcome them and lead a productive life. Actor Christopher Reeve became a quadriplegic after a fall from a horse. He has returned to acting. Franklin Roosevelt lost the use of his legs from polio and was subsequently elected to the presidency for 4 terms. And Lance Armstrong overcame testicular cancer to win the Tour de France. With your determination and the help of others, you will be able to lead a happy and successful life.

REFERENCES

Brown, Robert T., and Susan M. Coupey, editors. *Chronic and Disabling Disorders, Adolescent Medicine: State of the Art Reviews*. Philadelphia: Henley & Belfus, Inc., June 1994.

McAnarney, Elizabeth, Richard Kreipe, Donald Orr, and George Comerci, editors. *Textbook of Adolescent Medicine*. Philadelphia: W. B. Saunders Co., 1992.

Newacheck, P. W., M. A. McManus, and H. B. Fox. "Prevalence and Impact of Chronic Illness among Adolescents." *American Journal of Diseases of Children* 145 (December 1991): 1367–1373.

Pappas, Arthur M., editor. *Upper Extremity Injuries in the Athlete*. New York: Churchill Livingstone, 1995.

Index

Abdomen, 54, 81
Abrasion, 78
Abstinence, 46
Abstraction disability, 164
Academics, 153–54
Acculturation, 169
Acetazolamide, 122
Achilles tendinitis, 88
Acne, 16, 69, 95–96
Acquaintance rape, 59
Acquired Immunodeficiency Syndrome, 96, 186. *See also* HIV (Human Immunodeficiency Virus)
Acupressure, 138
Acupuncture, 138
Acute mountain illness, 122
Acyclovir, 51
Adam, 71
Adductor, 86
ADHD (Attention Deficit/Hyperactivity Disorder), 156
Adolescence, defined, xii
Africa, 135, 136
African American, 121, 170
Age, and sexually transmitted disease, 50
Aggression, 20, 21

AIDS (Acquired Immunodeficiency Syndrome), 96, 186. *See also* HIV (Human Immunodeficiency Virus)
Alcohol: and cold injuries, 118; and driving, 8–9; and drowning, 11; and high altitude, 122; and hypothermia, 117–18; and media, 22; and race, 170; reasons for use, 63–64; and sex, 45, 50, 57, 63, 176
Allergy, 96–97, 99, 131, 181, 182
Alopecia, 27, 97
Alternative medicine, 137–40
Altitude, 122
Amino acids, 40, 41
Amphetamines, 70
Anabolic steroids. *See* Steroids
Androstenedione, 40, 41–42
Anemia, 26, 27, 92
Angel dust, 72
Ankle, 88
Anorexia nervosa, 36
Anticholinergic reaction, 131
Anxiety disorder, 156–58
Apophysitis, of calcaneus, 88
Appetite, loss of, 54
Arch, 88
Arm, lower, 83

Aromatherapy, 138
Arthroscope, 87
Asia, 135, 136
Asthma, 76, 90–91, 97, 137–38, 181
Athlete. *See* Sports
Athlete's foot, 90
Attention Deficit Disorder, 156
Attention Deficit/Hyperactivity Disorder, 156
Autoimmune disorder, 100. *See also* Acquired Immunodeficiency Syndrome; Human Immunodeficiency Virus

Back, 89
Baldness, 69, 97
Barotitis media, 80
Barotrauma, 123
Baseball, 80, 82, 85, 90
Basketball, 78, 83–84, 88, 90
Bat bite, 130
Beans, 28
Bedwetting, 97
Bees, 126–27
Behavior: and hormones, 20–21; and nutrition, 151–52; and peers, 8–9; problems with, 162–63
Biking, 78, 80, 81, 92
Bipolar disorder, 155–56
Bites, 126, 129–31, 134
Black eye, 80
Blackfly, 127
Blackheads, 95
Black heel, 78
Black widow spider, 128–29
Bladder, 51
Blister, 77–78
Blood/bleeding: and blister, 78; and ejaculation, 100; and heat injury, 119; and sickle cell disease, 108; in urine, 81, 92, 101. *See also* Hypertension
Blood transfusion, and HIV, 55
Blotter acid, 70
BMI. *See* Body Mass Index
Body building. *See* Weight training
Body mass, 25

Body Mass Index, 32–33, 34
Body piercing, 98
Bodywork, 138–39
Bone, and syphilis, 53
Boxer's fracture, 85
Brain, and syphilis, 53. *See also* Nervous system
Breakfast, 152
Breakups, 147, 152, 160
Breast, development of, 19
Bronchospasm, 91
Brown recluse spider, 128
Bruise, 78
Burn, 123–24

Caffeine, 40, 41, 152
Calcaneus, apophysitis of, 88
Callus, 77
Calories, 26, 27, 30, 31, 33, 35
Cancer: dealing with, 181, 186; and genital warts, 54; and skin, 105; and sun, 120; and testicles, 110; tobacco as, 65
Carbohydrates, 27, 28, 37, 38, 39
Career, 23
Carnitine, 40, 41
Carpal tunnel syndrome, 85
CD (Conduct Disorder), 162–63
Celiac disease, 100
Centipede, 129
Chancre, 53
Cheese, 28
Chemical burn, 124
Chest, 80, 98
Chicken pox, 98
Chigger, 128
Chlamydia, 52–53
Chloroquine, 136
Cholera, 136
Cholesterol, 38, 98
Christian Scientists, 170
Chromium, 40–41
Chronic conditions, 181–87
Chronic fatigue syndrome, 99
Clavicle, 82
Closet, in the, 173
Clothing, outdoor, 117, 118, 119, 121

Cocaine, 67–68
Cold, and disease, 170–71
Cold, and injury, 118–19
Cold, common, 99
Cold fluid, 42
Cold-water immersion, 118–19
Coles, Robert, 45
Coming out, 173
Communication, 1–2, 5
Compliance, with physician, 5–6
Concussion, 78
Condom, 10, 45–47, 50, 96
Conduct Disorder, 162–63
Confidentiality, 2–3
Confusion, 72
Consciousness, loss of, 78, 101, 116
Consent, and physician, 3–4
Contraception, 46–49, 106
Control, 21
Coordination, and alcohol use, 63
Coping, 153, 160, 174
Corn, 77
Cornea, 118
Corn syrup, 28
Crabs, 54–55
Crack cocaine, 67
Creatine, 40
Crohn's disease, 104, 185
Cross-cultural issues, 169–71
Crotch, and crabs, 54–55
Crystalline methamphetamine, 70
Culture, 169
Cystic fibrosis, 99, 152

Date rape, 59
Date rape drug, 72–73
DDAVP, 97
Death, 11, 146–47, 160. *See also* Suicide
DEET, 127, 128
Dehydration, 39, 42–43
Delayed Onset Muscle Soreness, 93
Dental dam, 96
Depersonalization, 66–67
Depression, 27, 58, 67, 93, 152–56, 176, 185
Dermatitis, 99, 125, 126. *See also* Rash

Designer drugs, 71
DHEA, 40, 41
Diabetes, 35, 92, 99, 185–86
Diarrhea, 91, 100, 126, 133, 136
Diet, 100. *See also* Nutrition
Disability, 182
Discharge, at urination, 51, 52, 53
Disease: and culture, 170; and epidemiology, 7. *See also specific diseases*
Divorce, 146, 152
Dizziness, 72, 122
Dog bite, 130
Driving, 63, 64
Drowning, 11
Drowsiness, 72
Drugs: and depression, 152; and Human Immunodeficiency Virus, 55, 96; rates of use, 61–62; reasons for use, 61–62; and sex, 10, 45, 50, 176; and sexuality, 57; tobacco as, 65; and travel, 136–37
Dust, 72
Dysgraphia, 164

Ear, 80, 91, 123, 125, 182
Earlobe, 80
Eating disorder, 36
Ecstasy, 71
Education, 153–54, 164
Eggs, 28
EIA (Exercise-induced asthma), 76, 90–91
Ejaculation, bloody, 100
Elbow, 82–83
Electrical burn, 124
Electrolytes, 42
Elisa, 56
Emotions: and growth, 21–23; health of, 159–62; and masculinity, 36; and running, 93; and sexuality, 21
Endurance, 41
Enuresis, 97
Epidemiology, 7–12
Epididymis, 51
Epididymitis, 100
Estrogen, 41
Ethnic group, 169

Euphoria, 93
Europe, and alcohol use, 63
Exam, physical, 4, 5, 6
Exercise, 39; addiction to, 93; and asthma, 138; and heat injury, 119; and hematuria, 101; and hormones, 36; rates of, 10–11. *See also specific activities*
Exercise-induced asthma, 76, 90–91
Eye: protection of, 80, 118; yellowing of, 54

Fainting, 101
Famciclovir, 51
Fast food, 30–31
Fat, 28, 30, 38, 39
Fatigue, 67, 122
Fear, 157–58
Fever, 54, 98
Film. *See* Media
Finger, injury to, 85
Fire, 124
Fire ant, 126–27
Fish, 28
Flashback, 66, 70
Flea, 127
Flower remedy, 139
Fluid, 39, 42. *See also* Water
Follicle stimulating hormone, 15
Food. *See* Nutrition
Foot, 88–89
Football, 75, 82, 85, 86
Foreskin, 106
Fracture, 80
Frostbite, 118
Frostnip, 118
Fruit, 28
FSH. *See* Follicle stimulating hormone

Gangs, 163
Gastroesophageal reflux disease, 91
Gay adolescent, 57–58, 173–78
Gender identity, 173, 174
Genetics, 19, 33, 153, 178
Genital herpes, 51
Genitourinary tract, 81
GERD. *See* Gastroesophageal reflux disease

Giardia lamblia, 126
Gila monster, 130
Gingko biloba, 137
Glucose, 37
Glycogen, 37
Gonorrhea, 51 52
Groin, 54–55, 78, 81, 86, 104
Growing pains, 101
Growth: and hormone deficiency, 19; and nutrition, 25, 31–33; physical versus emotional, 15–23; and steroids, 69
Gums, 27
Gymnastics, 89

Hair, loss of, 27, 97
Hallucination, 67, 70, 71, 122
Hamstrings, 85
Hand, 85, 108
HDL cholesterol, 38
Head, injury to, 78–80
Headache, 93, 101, 136, 182
Healing touch, 138
Health, outdoor and wilderness, 115–31
Heart: and alcohol use, 63; and amphetamines, 70; disease of, 38; and heroin, 71; and syphilis, 53
Heat, 42–43, 119, 121, 170–71
Heat stroke, 42, 43
Heel, 78, 88
Height, 16–19, 31–32
Helmet, 7, 11, 78, 80
Hematuria, 81, 92, 101
Hemophilia, and Human Immunodeficiency Virus, 55
Hepatitis A, 102, 134, 135
Hepatitis B, 54, 102
Hepatitis C, 102
Herbal remedy, 137, 139
Hernia, 102
Heroin, 71
Herpes, genital, 51
Herpes gladiatorum, 76
Herpes simplex, 90
High altitude, 122
High blood pressure. *See* Hypertension

High water pressure, 122–23
Hip, 85–86
HIV (Human Immunodeficiency Virus), 55–57, 96, 175–76. *See also* Acquired Immunodeficiency Syndrome
Hockey, 78–79, 80, 86
Home, leaving, 147–48, 160
Homeopathy, 138
Homophobia, 57–58
Homosexuality, 57–58, 173–78
Hormones, 92; and acne, 95; and behavior, 20–21; and cholesterol, 38; and depression, 152; and diabetes, 99; and exercise, 36; and growth, 15, 19; and marijuana, 67; and puberty, 36; and sleep disorder, 160; treatment with, 15, 19; and weight, 33, 35
Hornet, 126
Human bite, 130–31
Human Immunodeficiency Virus, 55–57, 96, 175–76. *See also* Acquired Immunodeficiency Syndrome
Hydrocoele, 102
Hyperactivity, 156
Hypersomnia, 103
Hypertension, 103
Hyperthyroidism, 103
Hypoglycemia, 92
Hypothalmus, 15
Hypothermia, 115–16, 118, 121, 126
Hypothyroidism, 103
Hypoxia, 122

IBD (Inflammatory Bowel Disease), 100, 104, 185
IBS (Irritable Bowel Syndrome), 100
Identity, and sexuality, 21
Imipramine, 97
Immunization, 5, 133, 135
Imodium, 133
Impetigo, 103
Impotence, 103–4
Independence, 22, 147–48
Inflammatory Bowel Disease, 100, 104, 185
Inguinal hernia, 102

Inhalant, 72–73
Insomnia, 104
Insulin, 40, 41, 92, 99
Insurance, 171
Intestines, 91
Iron, 26, 151
Irritability, and cocaine, 67
Irritable Bowel Syndrome, 100
IV drug use, 55

Jaundice, 54
Jaw, 109
Jellyfish, 125
Jimsonweed, 131
Jock itch, 90, 104
Judgment, impaired, 116

Kidney calcium, 27
Kidneys, 38, 92, 186–87
Kidney stones, 27
Knee, 81–82, 86–87
Kyphosis, 104

Lacto-ovo-vegetarian, 27
Lacto-vegetarian, 27
Latin America, 135, 136
Latinos, 170–71
LDL cholesterol, 38
Learning disability, 164, 184
Leaving home, 147–48, 160
Leech, 125
Leg, 87–88
LH. *See* Luteinizing hormone
Lifting. *See* Weight training
Ligament, 86, 93
Lightning, 121–22
Light therapy, 139, 155
Little league elbow, 82
Liver, and Hepatitis B, 54
Lordosis, 104
LSD, 67, 70–71
Lungs, 90–91
Luteinizing hormone, 15
Lyme disease, 104–5, 128
Lysine, 41

Malaria, 136
Manic depression, 155–56

Marathon, 37, 38
Marijuana, 66–67
Masculinity, 21, 36, 58–59
Massage, 138, 139
Masturbation, 21, 105
MDMA, 71
Meat, 28
Media, 11–12, 22, 62, 142–43
Medial collateral ligament, 86
Medial meniscus, 86
Medicine, alternative, 137–40
Medicine, sports, 89–93
Meditation, 140
Mefloquine, 136
Melanoma, 105
Memory, 67, 72
Meningitis, 105
Meningococcal disease, 105, 135–36
Mental health, 9, 19, 70, 152–59, 170, 176–78. *See also specific problems*
Metatarsalgia, 89
Methionine, 41
Mexican beaded lizard, 130
Microdot, 70
Migraine. *See* Headache
Milk, 26, 27, 28
Millipede, 129
Minerals, 25, 26, 38
Minor: emancipated, 4; mature, 4
Minorities, 169
Monkeys, 134
Monogamy, 50
Mononucleosis, 81, 105–6
Mood, change in, 116
Morning after pill, 106
Mosquito, 127, 135
Mountain illness, 122
Mouth guard, 80
Mumps, 106
Muscle dysmorphia, 36
Muscles, 19, 40, 92–93
Mushrooms, 132

Native American, 170
Nausea, 54, 72, 93
Neck, injury to, 78–80
Needle, 134
Nervous system, 27, 63, 65, 70, 71, 93, 122, 152, 154

Neurofibromatosis, 184
Nicotine, 65
Night blindness, 27
Noise, 91
Nonoxynol 9, 47, 49
Nose, injury to, 79–80
Nutrition, 25–43, 151–52
Nutritional ergogenics, 40
Nuts, 28

Obesity, 33, 183–84
Obsessive-Compulsive Disorder, 156–57
OCD (Obsessive-Compulsive Disorder), 156–57
Oils, 28
Orchitis, 106
Osgood-Schlatter disease, 86
Osteochondritis dissecans, 87
Outdoors, 115–31
Oxygen, low levels of, 122

Pacific Rim countries, 136
Pain, at urination, 52
Panic, 66, 157–58
Papilloma virus, 54
Papules, 95, 106
Paranoia, 70
Parent: and alcohol use, 63; communication with, 5; and consent, 3–4; and drugs use, 62; and homosexuality, 58; and independence, 22; and physical exam, 4; relationship with, 23
Pasteurella multocida, 130
Patellofemoral syndrome, 86
PCP, 72
Peers, 8, 22, 62, 63
Penis, 51, 53, 106
Pepto-Bismol, 133
Perception, and LSD, 70
Perineum, 92
Permethrins, 127, 128
Perspiration, 42
Phimosis, 106
Phobia, 157–58
Phosphocreatine, 40
Physical activity. *See* Exercise
Physical exam, 4

Physician, relationship with, xii, 1–2, 6
Pickpocket, 136
Pink pearly penile papules, 106
Pit viper, 129–30
Place kicker, 85
Plantar fasciitis, 88
Plantar warts, 90, 106
Plants, dangers from, 131–32
Poison ivy, 126, 131
Poison oak, 131
Polysubstance abuse, 73
Portuguese man-of-war, 125
Post-traumatic stress Disorder, 156
Posture, 106. *See also* Spine
Poultry, 28
Poverty, 163
Prayer, 138
Preparticipation sports examination, 107
Preventive care, 107
Prostatitis, 107
Prostitution, 137; and cocaine, 68
Protein, 25, 26, 27, 37, 39; and kidneys, 38
Prozac, 154
Pseudoanemia, 92
Pseudomonas, 125
Psychosis, 72
Psychosomatic illness, 158
PTSD (Post-traumatic stress Disorder), 156
Puberty, 15–16; and hormones, 36
Pubic lice, 54–55
Pustules, 95

Quadriceps, 85

Rabies, 130, 134
Race, 163, 169, 170
Racquetball, 80
Rape, 12, 59, 72–73. *See also* Violence
Rash: and chicken pox, 98; and groin, 104; and Herpes gladiatorum, 76; and impetigo, 103; and Lyme disease, 104; and neurofibromatosis, 184; and plants, 131; and syphilis, 53. *See also* Dermatitis
Rat bite, 130

Reflexology, 140
Renal failure, 186–87
Repetitive strain injury, 107–8
Reptiles, 129–30
Respiration: and allergies, 181; and amphetamines, 70; and cystic fibrosis, 99; and heroin, 71; and high altitude, 122; injury to, 80; and malaria, 136; tobacco as, 66
Rickets, 27
Risk-taking, 21, 22
Ritalin, 156
Rocket fuel, 72
Rocky Mountain Spotted Fever, 128
Rohypnol, 72, 73
Role model, 22, 62
Roofies, 72–73
Rotator cuff, 82
Rugby, 85
Running, 37, 75–76, 87–88, 89, 91, 92, 93

Salmonella typhi, 135
Scald burn, 124
Schizophrenia, 70
School phobia, 157
School work, 153–54
Scoliosis, 108
Scorpion, 129
Scuba diving, 80, 91, 122–23
Seasonal affective disorder, 139, 154–55, 157
Sebum, 95
Seizure, 11, 70
Selective serotonin reuptake inhibitors, 154
Self-image, 22
Self-reliance. *See* Independence
Sequencing disability, 164
Setting, and physician, 2
Sex: and alcohol use, 45, 50, 57, 63, 176; and culture, 170; and drug use, 10; and homosexuality, 176; and Human Immunodeficiency Virus, 96; and marijuana, 67; and morning after pill, 106; oral, 45, 51; rates of, 10, 45; and travel, 137
Sex role, 173
Sexual abuse, 58–59, 161–62

Sexuality, 21, 45–59
Sexually transmitted disease, 3, 10, 45, 49–57, 175–76
Sexual orientation, 173
Shark, 124–25
Shin splints, 87–88
Shivering, 116, 118
Shoes, 88
Short-term memory disability, 164
Shoulder, 81
Sickle cell disease, 108
Skating, 84
Skin: and allergy, 182; and cancer, 105, 120; and hot tub, 125; and hypothermia, 116; and impetigo, 103; injuries to, 76–78, 90; and melanoma, 105; and neurofibromatosis, 184; problems with, 27; and rash, 53, 76, 98, 99, 103, 104, 125, 126, 131, 184; and sun, 120–21; and water sport, 125; yellowing of, 54
Skunk bite, 130
Sleep, 104, 152
Sleep disorder, 160
Sleepwalking, 108
Smoking, 22
Snakes, 129–30
Soccer, 85, 89
Sodium, 30
Solar health, 119–21
Speed, 41
Spermatocoele, 108
Spermicide, 47, 49
Spiders, 128–29
Spine, 104
Spleen, 81
Sports: examination for, 107; and injuries, 75–89; and marijuana, 67; and nutrition, 36–43; and steroids, 69; tobacco as, 66; water, 124–26; whitewater, 126. See also specific activities
Sports medicine, 89–93
Sprained ankle, 88
Squash, 80
SSRIs (Selective serotonin reuptake inhibitors), 154
Staph, 90, 103
Stature, 16–19

STD (Sexually transmitted disease), 3, 10, 45, 49–57, 175–76
Sterility, 106
Steroids, 36, 41, 68–69, 137, 152
Sting, 126, 127
Stingray, 125
Strep, 90, 103
Strep throat, 108
Stress, 95, 139, 140–42, 152, 160
Stretch marks, 76
Subluxation, 82
Subungual hematoma, 89
Sugar, 28, 37, 151–52
Suicide, 9–10, 58, 158–59, 176. See also Death
Sun, sensitivity to, 27
Sunburn, 119–20, 121, 126
Sunglasses, 121
Sunscreen, 119–20
Swimmer's ear, 125
Swimming, 11, 82, 134–35
Syphilis, 53
Syringe, 134

Tatoo, 108–9
Teeth, injury to, 80
Temporomandibular joint pain, 109
Tendinitis, 88
Tennis, 78, 80
Tennis elbow, 82–83
Testicle: and biking, 81; and hormones, 15; and orchitis, 106; and self-exam, 109–10; and steroids, 69; torsion of, 110; and tumor, 110; undescended, 111
Testosterone, 15–16, 19, 41–42, 68
THC, 66
Thermoregulation, 121. See also Cold; Heat; Hypothermia
Thigh, 85–86
Thorn, 131
Thyroid, 35
Tick, 104, 105, 128
Time-management skills, 142
Tinea crucis, 90
TM (Temporomandibular joint pain), 109
Tobacco, 64–66, 122

Toe, 89
Toenail, 78, 89
Tofranil, 97
Transient neurologic impairment, 78
Trauma, 156
Traumatic hematuria, 81, 92, 101
Travel, 133–48
Traveler's diarrhea, 133
TSE (Testicular self-exam), 109–10
Turf toe, 89
Typhoid, 135

Ulcerative colitis, 104
Ultraviolet light, 119, 121
Unconsciousness, 78, 101, 116
Urethra, 51
Urethritis, 111
Urine, 51, 52, 53, 81, 92, 101

Vaccination. See Immunization
Valacyclovir, 51
Vampire bat, 130
Varicoele, 111
Vegan, 27
Vegetables, 28
Vegetarian, 27
Vertebra, 89
Violence, 142–45, 163; and aggression, 21; and homosexuality, 173, 174; and LSD, 70; and media, 11–12; and school, 9; and women, 12. See also Rape

Visual disturbance, 72, 93
Vitamin B6, 137
Vitamins, 25, 26, 27, 38
Vomiting, 72, 93

Warts, 54, 90, 106
Wasp, 126–27
Water: and cholera, 136. See also Fluid
Water, contaminated, 134–35
Water, intake of, 42
Water, retention of, 40
Water pressure, 122–23
Weapons, and school, 9
Weight, 16–19, 25, 32, 33–36, 38–39
Weight training, 19, 37, 38, 69, 93
Western Blot, 56
Whitewater sports, 126
Wilderness, 115–31
Wind, 121
Windowpane, 70
Withdrawal, 46, 71
Women, 12, 21, 22
Work, 163
Wrestling, 39, 76, 82, 90
Wrist, injury to, 83–84, 108
Wrist guard, 84

Yellow fever, 135
Yoga, 138
Yogurt, 28

Zoloft, 154

About the Authors

MARK A. GOLDSTEIN, M.D. is an adolescent healthcare specialist.

MYRNA CHANDLER GOLDSTEIN is an independent scholar and free-lance writer.